Biological, Chemical, and Nuclear Warfare

Protecting Yourself
and Your Loved Ones:
The Power of Digital Medicine

Savely Yurkovsky, M.D.

Science of Medicine Publishing
Chappaqua, New York

Published by
Science of Medicine Publishing
37 King Street
Chappaqua, NY 10514
e-mail: Books@ScienceOfMedicinePublishing.com
website: www.ScienceOfMedicinePublishing.com

Printed in the United States of America.

FIRST EDITION

Library of Congress Cataloging-in-Publication Data is available upon request.
Yurkovsky, Savely
Biological, Chemical, and Nuclear Warfare. Protecting Yourself and Your Loved
Ones: The Power of Digital Medicine / Savely Yurkovsky.

Includes bibliographical references and index.
ISBN 0-9726346-0-6 (pbk.).

Library of Congress Control Number: 2002115966

Cover by Eric Elias.
Book design by ATLIS Graphics.

To all the victims of September 11,
their families, and rescue workers.

Acknowledgements

This author is grateful to his office staff members: Jankie Whittaker, Franka Constantinou, and Eileen Ford for their years of diligent work on the manuscript and especially to Esther Baltunis for her tenacity, patience and dedication. Thanks also to Diane Ford and Debbie Jacobs for their assistance with office work.

Much appreciation is extended to Kristin Nord for fine editing.

Deep gratitude to Professor Emeritus of Stanford University, William A. Tiller, for his guidance concerning the scientific aspects of this book.

Acknowledgement is emphatically due to my wife and my children for their sacrifices, to my parents, my brother, and Elfriede and Walter Schoendorf for their support.

Disclaimer and note to the reader

Some of the medical methods proposed in this book aimed at alleviation of the consequences of biological, toxicological or nuclear warfare may not constitute "standard medical practice." Consult your physician for advice.

In order to protect the identity of the patients' cases presented in this book, names have been changed as well as other identifying characteristics.

Contents

Chapter 10   A Brief Analysis of the Benefits and Limitations of the Main Homeopathic Approaches in Cases of Biological, Toxicological and Nuclear Warfare   133

Chapter 11   Anthrax and its Homeopathic and Conventional Management   139

Chapter 12   Smallpox and its Homeopathic and Conventional Management   155

Chapter 13   Other Supportive Measures and Considerations   167

Chapter 14   Post Traumatic Stress Syndrome and Psychological Problems Following September 11th   173

"Most diseases can be cured through the very same factors in which they originate."

Hippocrates

Foreword

Savely Yurkovsky, M.D., has provided us with a remarkable and timely book that will greatly assist world populations in effectively dealing with the multitude of personal health challenges to be faced as a consequence of both (1) continuing terrorist activities within national boundaries and (2) the growing toxicological side-effects associated with our chemical, pharmaceutical and electromagnetic industries. His well-founded advice is based upon his long-standing community service experience as a homeopathic medical practitioner who also is highly expert in the use of the "Bio-resonance Diagnostic Technique". Not only does he provide us with abundant medical case histories from his own office files and also from widespread publications around the world but he shows us how to quickly and cheaply make remedies for ourselves, our families and our neighbors from the products of our own bodies after they have responded to the multiple stressors generated by nearby or distant terrorist attacks.

One century ago, the number of homeopathic medical practitioners in the USA and Europe was rapidly growing and catching up with the numbers of allopathic (conventional medical) practitioners. However, the physical science studies of the past century have almost completely focused on the coarse chemical particulate level of physical reality and this experimental data greatly buttressed the allopathic viewpoint to the detriment of the homeopathic viewpoint. Profit-driven professional rivalries plus pharmaceutical corporate greed led to the demise of those colleges devoted to homeopathy training so that by the middle of the past century there were very few practicing homeopathic MDs. However, for the past few decades, their numbers have been growing by leaps and bounds.

One reason for this has been the availability of new tools by which to conduct of detailed experiments in the areas of subtle energies and energy medicine. Another has been the disenchantment of the general public with both the cost, marginal effectiveness and unwanted side-effects associated with allopathic or "chemical" medicine.

To illustrate the key difference in these two levels of medical understanding, let me use the following example. It is well known that placing colloidal particles of silver into a beaker of water that contains bacteria will kill the bacteria. What is not so well known is that placing these colloidal silver particles in a nearby gas discharge tube, and focusing the electromagnetic emissions from such an operating tube onto the beaker, will also kill the bacteria. Thus, physical contact between the bacteria and the silver is not a **necessary** condition for killing the bacteria. Further, if one looks at the optical spectrum of silver and then combines the magnitudes of the optical output for several light sources of different frequencies so as to closely simulate the silver spectrum, such a beam of electromagnetic radiation will also kill these bacteria. Via this simple example we see that it is **the specific information pattern** inherent in the silver atom and not the physical contact that is killing the bacteria. And our general present-day experience with transforming one computer language to another shows us that the same basic information pattern (the same meaning) can exist in many different formats. Thus, to understand the homeopathic/allopathic medicine duality, we must focus our attention on the various possible information pattern formats that Nature utilizes to express itself.

Dr. Yurkovsky refers to my two recent books, where one can explore some of the details behind my following statements, so I will utilize simple "bullet-type" assertions concerning my present views on how Nature expresses itself in what we call "physical reality":

- De Broglie, in the 1920's, provided us with the concept that every particle in Nature traveled with its own pilot wave envelope around it. This became a cornerstone of present-day quantum mechanics.
- The primary waves making up such an envelope were ultimately labeled **information waves** because they traveled at velocities greater than the speed of light.

- Recent experiments strongly suggest that (1) magnetic monopoles, functioning at the vacuum level between the fundamental particles that comprise atoms and molecules, "write" these information waves, (2) a coupling substance (labeled deltrons) from the higher dimensional domain of emotion allows the coarse electric particles and these fine information waves to interact so as to provide electromagnetism (EM); and (3) human intention is able to interact directly with the deltrons so as to change the degree of this EM coupling and alter the magnitude of physical measurement.
- The magnitude of any physical measurement, and thus what we call physical reality, is comprised of two parts: (1) the coarse particulate part; and (2) the fine information wave part. The magnitude of the second part is small relative to the first in our normal cognitive reality; however, it can be made larger using special procedures.
- The information wave aspect of Nature is the precursor template for the coarse particulate aspect so that manipulation of this aspect can have significant influence on the structure and functionality of the coarse particulate aspect.
- Thus, in the above example of silver and the bacteria, manipulating the information aspect of the silver can alter the information aspect of the bacteria in such a way as to "kill" the bacteria entity.
- Homeopathy is thought to act on the information wave aspect of a particular remedy rather than the coarse particulate aspect (where allopathy reigns) and thus can display powerful medical therapeutic action on all life forms.
- Finally, quantitative mathematics connecting the fine information wave domain of Nature with the coarse particulate domain of Nature shows that the **total** thermodynamic activity of a particular remedy, "j", in an aqueous solution can continue to increase during the succussion/dilution process even when the coarse particulate concentration of "j" falls below the Avogadro number limit.

What we begin to see here in this homeopathic/allopathic duality is Nature expressing itself via what is beginning to look like a hierarchy of information patterns. Allopathic procedures and techniques have taught us a great deal about the coarse particulate patterns of the hierarchy while homeopathy, acupuncture and advanced kinesiology (with its Bio-resonance diagnostic technique) are beginning to teach us a great deal about the fine information wave patterns of this information hierarchy. Dr. Yurkovsky's wonderful spectrum of case studies again and again bring home the power of carefully applied homeopathic knowledge for restoring balance and health to important aspects of the human body. I have learned a great deal from this book, it has significantly enhanced my perspective concerning the homeopathy/allopathy modalities of treatment and relative benefits and it taught me a cardinal rule concerning the role of a human observer: "Pay attention to the experimental data, no matter how confounding it is to current theoretical models of Nature." This book shows us an abundance of experiential data in support of the view that allopathic medical understanding is only the tip of the iceberg concerning the totality of medical understanding. Dr. Yurkovsky is to be congratulated on this fine contribution to help us "see the light" and for showing us relatively simple pathways to protect and treat ourselves from the various traumatic stressors that appear to be part of our near future.

Professor Emeritus of Materials Science,
William A. Tiller, Stanford University
Author *"Science and Human Transformation: Subtle Energies, Intentionality and Consciousness"*

Preface

The catastrophic events following September 11th, 2001, have vividly revealed to all of us the vast inadequacy of conventional medicine (the medical system that has monopolized our health care) to handle the broad range of medical consequences in the event of terrorist attacks.

Millions of New York City residents, including thousands of the heroic workers at "Ground Zero," were exposed to a vast array of toxic pollutants as a result of the collapse of the World Trade Center Towers. These pollutants included asbestos, mercury, burnt plastics, fiberglass and other carcinogenic substances. Many "Ground Zero" workers, including firemen and police officers, developed serious respiratory ailments and now face various degrees of permanent disability. The long-term health implications of exposure to these noxious pollutants are impossible to predict because of the severe limitations of conventional diagnostic methods, yet they are expected to be very significant and to include increased cancer rates.

In addition to terrorist-induced exposure to pollutants, respiratory anthrax, spread through the postal system, killed as many as 50% of those who were infected. This high percentage of deaths occurred despite the fact that all of the infected patients were treated with the super powerful and costly antibiotic, Cipro, reputed to be the best therapy conventional medicine has to offer against this fatal disease. Given these results, it is clear that the tolls of biological, toxicological, or nuclear terrorism will be astronomical should future attacks occur.

U.S. government officials have openly admitted the inevitability of even worse terrorist attacks against the general civilian population as the war against Iraq proceeds. One needs only to ask: "What would I do—what *could* I do, in the face of a terrorist attack that employs methods of mass destruction? What would I do to protect my children, my spouse, myself?" to realize that as a nation, we are frighteningly under-equipped for the actuality of such an event.

The emotional terror in the aftermath of the tragedy of September 11th, as well as the chain of threats that forecast additional terrorist attacks, sent millions of frightened individuals across the nation into a state of frenzy. The demand for anti-anxiety drugs, sleeping pills and coping medications skyrocketed, notwithstanding their cost, multiple side effects, and consequent chemical dependency. Most importantly, these psychotropic interventions fail to offer true healing to the afflicted.

The environmental hazards at "Ground Zero" were more clearly revealed on December 11, 2001, when the Fox Channel's *The O'Reilly Factor* examined the progressive health deterioration of the rescue workers there. One fireman on the program voiced his feelings of hopelessness and despair at becoming a chronic invalid with a diminished lifespan. Similarities with the workers' plight and with that of our veterans afflicted with the mysterious Gulf War Syndrome seemed sadly appropriate.

Another guest on the program, a conventional medical doctor from a prestigious university hospital in New York City, was unable to offer much hope and only promised to "watch" the workers. Because conventional medicine is capable neither of effectively identifying the toxic substances that have invaded the internal organs nor of removing them, the promise to "watch" has only one practical meaning: to observe passively each person's physical destruction while busily performing the myriads of tests which document the downhill course.

Despite the obvious and severe limitations in the ability of conventional medicine to handle these crises, no serious attempts have been made to incorporate other medical options. Alternative and integrative forms of medicine have been grossly underutilized, despite their potential to provide better, safer, and more economical options. Much of this is due to a generally accepted presumption that alternative medicine represents inferior science. This blanket dismissal of integrative and alternative medicine has reduced them to the status of medical orphans. Yet, as this book will demonstrate, the presumption of inferior science does not withstand rigorous impartial scientific scrutiny. Rather, it is based upon cultural myth. The myth of the inferiority of alternative medicine is an unavoidable psychological by-product in a society preoccupied with body chemistry-based approaches. This overall commitment has propelled staggering financial rewards for the pharmaceutical industry and related research sector, and monopolized healthcare to the exclusion and suppression of other more effective and much less costly approaches to wellness.

The purpose of this book is to share with the reader the great body of compelling alternative scientific and clinical evidence that is indeed available. I welcome the reader to rediscover, through these pages, the most powerful therapeutic system in the world— *Homeopathy.* This approach, guided by Bio-resonance testing, is capable of identifying within seconds the biological, chemical or radioactive agents that are deposited within the body. Homeopathy acts precisely, on a deep and fundamental dimension of human physiology: the energy fields of our cells.

I invite the reader to explore in these pages the ways in which homeopathy and Bio-resonance testing offer superior medical interventions in accordance with the established standards of science. Because they act upon physiologic pathways through extraction and delivery of precise energetic information, they can be considered *digital medical* interventions.

It is not widely appreciated within the chemistry-based medical paradigm that profound changes in the body can be triggered through precision medicines, which act as signals on energetic aspects of our human physiology. Because immune and detoxifying organs charged with combating biological and chemical assaults possess these energetic aspects, too, they are able to be turned on by these signals and act against specific noxious agents promptly and efficiently. Based upon this principle, homeopathic digital vaccines and antidotes can be produced against any agent of terror aimed at the destruction of Man. Furthermore, *these preventatives and cures can be produced easily and within minutes by anyone.* Moreover, these energetic therapeutics offer an unsurpassed versatility—they can be prepared just as rapidly against unexpected or mutated strains of biological pathogens for which no conventional vaccines even exist. Their action is powerful and rapid while their cost is miniscule and their side-effects, if any, are rare and few.

The information presented in this book offers potentially life-saving skills to readers and their loved ones. These methods can be used with equal benefit in cases of epidemic, industrial or household environmental contamination, or nuclear accidents.

Due to the serious nature of the subject involved, it is incumbent upon the author to include the body of data presenting scientific evidence in its support. Some readers, understandably, may find some of the material technical. However, all readers stand to benefit greatly from the self-help section and by familiarizing themselves with the many clinical cases—and attendant cures—that demonstrate the unparalleled efficacy of this medical system.

Chapter 1

What is Homeopathy, How Did it Come About and What Are Its Methods?

The term "homeopathy" originates from the Greek words *homoeos* (similar) and *pathos* (pathology or disease). Unlike allopathy or conventional medicine, which applies means that are antagonistic or opposite to disease, homeopathic cures use the very substances which, given to a healthy person, are capable of producing the same disease or ailment. In case of a fever, the allopathic approach would indicate suppressing the fever through anti-fever drugs. Homeopathy would administer a remedy that would *produce* fever in a healthy person.

The founder of homeopathy, the German physician Samuel Hahnemann, MD (1755–1843), made an interesting observation in 1791. He conducted an unusual experiment, in an attempt to determine why extracts of Peruvian Bark *(Cinchona officinalis),* from which the drug quinine is made, were so effective in the treatment of one of the worst malaria epidemics of his time. Hahnemann began administering the bark extract to himself, hoping that by experiencing its taste and other properties he would be able to gain a better understanding of its therapeutic effect. To his astonishment, he discovered that he began to experience the symptoms of the very disease that the bark was supposed to cure—malaria itself. Hahnemann realized that this was not just an accident. He had discovered a phenomenon with tremendous medicinal potential.

As far back as the fifth century BC, Hippocrates, the "Father of Medicine," had promoted the seemingly eccentric therapeutic principle known as "like cures like." Later, the theory was explored further by the great Swiss physician, Theophrastus Paracelsus. Hahnemann extended this principle to a much deeper level and wider application. He undertook a systematic study of numerous known toxins by administering them to himself, his family members and other healthy volunteers, but in a very diluted form in order to avoid triggering significantly harmful effects. Hahnemann meticulously recorded the symptoms that he and the volunteers experienced. Later, he administered to his patients those substances that had produced similar symptoms in healthy volunteers. He began observing marked improvement in many conditions otherwise considered to be incurable at the time. Hahnemann summarized his observations and experience in the *Law of Similars*.

He noticed, however, that after a certain amount of dilution, substances lost their therapeutic power. Then, for reasons he never revealed, he began complementing every step of dilution by delivering a certain number of mechanical impacts against the bottoms of the vials containing the diluted substance. Oddly enough, this step resulted in a tremendous increase in the therapeutic effectiveness of the new remedies. Paradoxically, their effectiveness continued to increase with each subsequent dilution/impact cycle during processing. (The mechanisms of action of homeopathic remedies will be discussed later.)

The paradoxes of Hahnemann's system, however, did not end with treating the ill with the "like cures like" principle and with over-diluted medicines that contained virtually undetectable traces of the original substance; rather, they proceeded from another, seemingly intuitive observation. In the choice of a remedy, the more common features of a disease were less important than the unusual and *peculiar* features.

Furthermore, no matter how deeply any disease process has engaged the corporal body, a treating physician must always take into consideration the complete psychosomatic features of an *individual*. He must pay special attention to the patient's emotions, state of mind and general body characteristics as well as the disease's specific features.

The physician would gather the following information for diagnosis and treatment:

• **Familial**—genetic predispositions
• **Triggering factors**—what preceded the onset of illness: physical or emotional injury; prolonged periods of stress; exposure to ele-

ments such as heat, cold, wind or rain; overindulgence in food, alcohol or sex; exposure to infectious or toxicological agents

- **Onset of an illness**—sudden and rapidly progressing or slow and gradual
- **Physical appearance**—pale or red, bloated or besotted, toxic or normal
- **Mental-Emotional state**—anxious and fearful or lethargic and indifferent; wanting company or to be left alone; pleading to be taken immediately to a doctor or screaming at the doctor to get away; hysterical, hypochondriacal or stoical
- **General**—hot or cold; perspiration/discharges—absent or present—their character, intensity, odor; thirsty, hungry or not thirsty and without appetite; periodicity of illness: weekly, monthly, or seasonally
- **Overall reaction to pathology**—to gauge the individual's underlying body-energy force and reserve—sluggish, intense, intermediate
- **Modalities** (factors that improve or worsen the state of an *individual*): sensitivity to light or darkness, noise or silence, warm or cool air, smell, and preferred temperature of liquids or foods

The main reason for such a detailed analysis is to create a total or as nearly perfect a match as possible between the many characteristics and general energy states of both a *remedy* and the ill *person*. Otherwise, if a "flu remedy" that is "hot, rapid and intense" is administered to a person who is "cold, slow and sluggish," the remedy will not be capable of eliciting the desired reaction, that of normalizing the ill body's pathological energetic imbalance.

The *Law of Totality,* which is based on this total match, is one of the *Laws of Cure* described by Hahnemann.[1] All of the characteristics and indications of each of the hundreds of homeopathic remedies were determined by *provings*—hundreds or even thousands of symptoms elicited in large groups of healthy volunteers who took an individual remedy.

Unusual or peculiar characteristics that present as symptoms are not a normal part of a generic disease condition. For example, if a person afflicted with pneumonia begins to experience a skin itch or a fear of ghosts, these characteristics would not normally constitute a part of the pathological picture pertaining to infection in the lungs. Yet, as Hahnemann astutely perceived, such characteristics are at least as important as the degree of a fever, or the nature of cough or sputum. It is through these unusual characteristics that the body reveals its inner workings and the weaknesses of an individual's entire defense system. Once the correct remedy is administered, the body's inherent defenses will be able to receive from the remedy the missing signal that will trigger and properly channel the body's untapped reserves. The recruitment of these reserves will allow the ill person to overcome the pathology and return to health.

Two hundred years ago, Hahnemann's medical system, which refused to confine the complex workings of a human being merely to the anatomic borders of his organs, struck his allopathic colleagues as quite eccentric. It remains just as incomprehensible to the majority of conventional allopathic doctors today. Yet in those years, scientific discoveries have confirmed the countless intricate interconnections and relationships upon which Hahnemann's system of preventive and therapeutic medicine is based.[2-5] Hahnemann's very detailed approach, based upon the totality of a person and the *Law of Similars,* is known as *classical homeopathy.*

Another classical homeopathic methodology is *genus epidemicus,* which applies in particular to severe epidemics or to biological warfare. This approach also is based on the analysis of the characteristics of an illness, and seeks to determine the "average" characteristics and symptoms of a group of individuals stricken by a given epidemic. The reason for this focus is two-fold. When the offending agent is highly virulent and has a very strong affinity for certain organs and tissues, the majority of affected persons (at least initially) can be expected to show common reactions. For example, most patients infected with cholera will develop a pattern of continuous watery diarrhea with incessant rectal contractions, leading to dehydration and vascular collapse. Similarly, burn victims will share such characteristics as severe swelling, large blisters, pain, and restlessness. Based upon an understanding of the shared characteristics of reactions to an epidemic or disaster, an experienced homeopath may select a remedy that will be effective either as the treatment (at least at the initial stages) of the epidemic, for the injury caused by the disaster, or as a prophylaxis for the majority of unaffected people.

Isopathy is another approach used in homeopathy; it follows the principle "the same cures the same." Isopathy is based upon the knowledge of which noxious factor is producing an illness. Whether it is an infectious, toxicological, nuclear or other disease-producing agent, it will be treated by administering the same agent in homeopathic form. The main proponent of isopathy was a German homeopath and professor of veterinary medicine, Wilhelm Lux, who created the first vaccine against anthrax in homeopathic form after extracting it from the diseased spleen tissue of an infected sheep. Homeopathic remedies prepared from noxious agents are called *isodes* (some call them *nosodes*) and are administered to neutralize the same agents in the patient.

An offshoot of the isopathic approach is *autoisopathy,* a method wherein remedies called *autoisodes* are prepared directly from bodily fluids—blood, saliva, urine, pus or other discharges—which usually contain the disease-producing agents themselves and their toxic by-products. As an example, bacteria such as staphylococcus or anthrax cause damage not only via their direct invasion but also through the secretion of special toxins that can cause even more damage to the infected person than the bacterial load itself. Thus, body fluids represent an ideal medium for containing these toxic elements and rendering them effective as homeopathic antidotes.

This branch of homeopathy, which deals with the administration of causative agents, isodes or autoisodes, can be classified as *causative homeopathy.* Unlike classical homoeopathy, causative homeopathy aims its prescriptions solely against the offending agents rather than the symptoms produced by these agents.

There are also *complex remedies,* which combine several individual remedies, and may include preparations of causative agents, such as several strains of influenza virus, or a mixture of toxicological agents, such as asbestos, carbon monoxide, pesticides or other environmental pollutants. Complex remedies may also contain several classical homeopathic remedies.

In the following sections, several clinical examples will illustrate the application of these methods.

Classical Homeopathy

Some years ago I received a very disturbing phone call from a patient of mine, Mr. B., an energetic and successful businessman. Departing from his normally upbeat and macho demeanor, he was crying into the phone like a baby. Knowing his personality well, I assumed some personal tragedy had taken place. Fortunately, I was wrong. Mr. B. told me that a few weeks earlier he had come down with an insidious flu, which began with a low-grade fever, watery sinus discharge, and feelings of sluggishness. He did not bother seeking help, expecting to shake off the "lousy bug" on his own by using various cold pills and liquids from his medicine chest. However, relief did not come; in fact, he just got sicker and sicker. By the time he contacted me, he had become very weak and completely listless—an enervated physical state that was totally uncharacteristic of him. He felt overwhelmed by inexplicable depression and anxiety, a sense of despondency and impending doom, as if something terrible were going to happen to him. His mind had become dull and he could not figure out why he had lost control of his senses and his life so rapidly. He was not thirsty, was bothered by light; yet sitting in the dark made his fears even more intolerable, causing a tremor in his hands. An added concern was that his secretary appeared to be suffering from the same depression, following a similar episode of flu two months before. Although her cold symptoms had abated, her depression had not and she was now taking antidepressant drugs and being treated by a psychiatrist on a regular basis. Mr. B. did not wish to resort to either of these options, but he didn't know what else to do.

His illness was characterized by these disease features:

- Insidious onset with low fever
- Slow progression
- Muscular weakness with tremor and fatigue
- Severe depression with sense of impending doom
- Despair with irrational anticipatory fear
- Anxiety about the future
- In doubt of recovery as manifested by the fear of remaining ill and requiring psychiatric care
- Watery nasal discharge
- Lack of thirst
- Sensitivity to both presence and deprivation of light

In the field of toxicology, the study of poisons, it is known that all of these effects are experienced when a person becomes poisoned with the toxic alkaloids contained in *Gelsemium sempervirens,* a plant native to North America commonly known as yellow jasmine.

It was obvious that, considering his gradual course, he required a *similar* remedy which would produce sluggish and slowly evolving symptoms if given to healthy individuals. In addition, it would have to have an affinity for the central and peripheral nervous systems since Mr. B's state of depression and tremor were pointing in these directions. Therefore, I administered a high potency homeopathic form of *Gelsemium sempervirens.* Mr. B recovered completely and rapidly without requiring psychiatric care or psychotropic drugs. In summary, even though Mr. B. had never actually ingested the toxic yellow jasmine plant, his disease features resembled those caused by its toxic effects, and the homeopathic remedy elicited the desired response on the part of his defense system.

Causative Homeopathy

Mrs. M. was experiencing the symptoms of a common cold during a winter flu epidemic. She complained of a sore throat, sinus congestion, sneezing, a fever of 102°F, muscle aches, headache and general malaise. It was obvious that she had caught a flu virus. The homeopathic isode flu virus preparation, *Influenzinum,* administered once in medium potency *30C,* seemed to have neutralized the "bug." Within 48 hours, her symptoms were gone.

Autoisodes

The pneumonia epidemic in England and Scotland following World War II was accompanied by an extremely toxic blood infection, *septicemia,* which claimed many lives. Often, these patients were brought to hospitals at a late and far advanced stage and were too ill to give the treating homeopathic physicians much of the information needed to find the correct classical remedy. Under these circumstances, remedies were prepared from the patients' own blood and then administered. This proved to be very effective and only rarely was a second or third dose necessary.[6]

Complex Homeopathy

A patient of mine complained of severe headaches, high blood pressure, flushed face, insomnia and chemical sensitivity. Her symptoms began after her neighbors sprayed their lawn with pesticides. She tried allopathic drugs, vitamins and acupuncture without much success. A complex remedy containing several kinds of homeopathically prepared pesticides, taken once, cleared all of her symptoms.

Homeopathy—The Least Understood Medical System: Answers to Common Questions

Historically, homeopathy has been the least understood medical system, posing by far the greatest conceptual challenges even to many health professionals. It is important at this juncture to address a number of issues that skeptics find very puzzling and commonly but erroneously use to discredit homeopathy.

Q: What sense does it make to give a patient more of the same poison that is making him ill in the first place, e.g., asbestos, lead, smallpox or anthrax? This seems irrational and dangerous. How can it possibly help anyone?
A: Homeopathic remedies contain barely detectable amounts of these noxious agents. In their higher dilutions and greater potencies they usually do not contain any of the original substance, but only its energetic printout.

Q: How are homeopathic medicines prepared?
A: All homeopathic remedies are created from the original substance in its crude form: any substance existing in Nature or encountered in the daily environment. Even substances or entities of relatively immaterial nature such as sun rays, x-rays, electric or magnetic fields, and ionizing radiation can form the basis for homeopathic remedies when brought into contact with water media.

In the preparation of a homeopathic medicine, an original substance, such as a plant, viral culture, or other, is usually placed in a solution of alcohol and water. The alcohol, however, is required only if a solid substance needs to be dissolved. It is also used as a preservative by homeopathic pharmacies, but its presence is not necessary for the therapeutic action. For home preparation, alcohol will not be needed; indeed, some people might be allergic to it.

After the basic solution is prepared, one drop of it is transferred into a glass vial containing 99 drops of water. Following this dilution, the therapeutic potency of a remedy is increased by a vigorous mechanical agitation (succussion) of the solution between twenty to forty times. This can be performed with a mechanical device delivering impacts to the bottom of the vial or by striking the vial against a relatively hard surface such as a book, hand, or even a carpeted floor. Therapeutic efficacy will be adequate even after ten succussions.

A remedy prepared after this first cycle, consisting of one dilution process and a single series of mechanical agitations, between 20 and 40 succussions, is assigned the homeopathic potency of 1C. "C" stands for *Centesimal,* reflecting a 1:100 dilution process.

After a 1C potency has been made, the preparation process is repeated in the same manner. One drop of 1C solution is added to 99 drops of water in another vial. Following the same number of mechanical agitations, the potency rises one step higher to 2C. This process can be repeated many times, up to thousands, tens of thousands and even a million or more times in order to have the same remedy available in a wide variety of potencies.

When the potency or dilution reaches a multiple of a thousand, the letter "M" is used to represent one thousand potency (a total dilution of $1:100^{1,000}$). In other words, 1000C is expressed as 1M, 10,000C as 10M, and so on. When the dilution reaches 100,000C, an extremely high potency, it is expressed as CM, and a 1,000,000C potency as MM, reflecting that a 1:100 dilution was carried out sequentially one hundred thousand and one million times (a total dilution of $1:100^{1,000,000}$), correspondingly. Homeopathic remedies that are prepared using smaller sequential dilutions of 1:10 each, i.e., 1 drop of solution per 9 drops of water, using the same serial mechanical agitation process, are represented by the letter "X", or in Europe, by the letter "D."

Another way of preparing homeopathic remedies is called Korsakov's Method, which will be presented later in this book. The potencies of the remedies prepared by this method are expressed by the letter "K".

From the pure rules of chemical dilutions that keep count of a number of parts of a substance remaining in a certain volume of dilutant with each sequential dilution, not even a single molecule of an original substance is expected to remain after dilutions above 12C (a total dilution of $1:100^{12}$) or 24X (a total dilution of $1:10^{24}$— "*Avogadro's number*"). Yet, the greater the dilution, the higher the potency, the stronger a remedy becomes.

There are four general therapeutic categories of potency strength:

Low:

1X	3X	6X	9X	12X	15X
1C	3C	6C	9C	12C	
1K	3K	6K	9K	12K	15K

Medium:

30X	60X	200X
15C	30C	60C
30K	60K	200K

High:
200C ; 1M, 10M—in X or C or K.

Very high:
50M, 100M—in X or C or K.

In rare circumstances, even higher potencies may be prepared.

It is imperative that high potency remedies are to be administered with caution and only by those with solid professional training.

Emphasis should be made that under the proper storage conditions, homeopathic remedies, regardless of their mode of preparation, remain efficacious indefinitely. Preparations sold commercially are usually required to display an expiration date, but this is a mere formality. Homeopathic remedies are capable of remaining potent for decades.

Q: The preparation process seems to produce medicines that are practically devoid of anything. How could such medicines, which become virtually nothing more than pure water, possibly act?
A: First of all, it is not a prerequisite for medicines to contain a material substance in order to promote healing effects. Such a requirement is necessary only for *pharmaceutical medicines,* whose action is based on the principles of chemistry because they are measured and dispensed in units of weight: grams, milligrams or even micrograms. This category includes pharmaceutical drugs, herbs, vita-

mins, nutritional supplements, aromatic oils and others. The effects of these substances on the body depend upon their chemical properties and their concentration within the body.

However, the human body also can be affected by many other factors in Nature that do not represent pharmaceutical or chemical agents *per se*. Instead, these factors represent energetic forces that are capable of acting at the level of our *energy body*. For example, we all know how simple words delivered as bad news may put a person in a state of shock, hysteria or cause a stroke, heart attack, mental breakdown or even death. Likewise, kind words, happy news, positive emotions are known to enhance our health significantly. Factors such as heat or cold may produce opposite effects on our physiology. Certain color spectra or musical sounds also affect us. The moon or the sun's rays affect our psyche and health as well. Statistics confirm that many people experience mental-emotional instability even to the point of committing crimes, suffering convulsions or cardiovascular events during geomagnetic fluctuations.[7–11] More commonly, tens of millions of people are known to be affected by SAD (Seasonal Affective Disorder) and become severely depressed and ill when deprived of exposure to sunlight during the winter months.

The Chinese Qi Gong therapy (which involves a transfer of positive energy from a therapist to a patient), acupuncture, medical visualization, reflexology, bio-feedback, and other methods are among numerous examples of non-pharmaceutical therapies that can offer significant health benefits. In fact, the most miraculous and baffling recoveries, examined from the standpoint of conventional chemico-pharmaceutical medicine, have taken place over many centuries following the laying on of hands or resulting from prayer whose benefits have reached patients from a far distance.[12]

All of these therapies or practices are energetic in nature and most of their actions can be explained through physics. The evidence of healing they offer clearly conflicts with the long-entrenched belief, rooted in materialistic pharmaceutical medicine, that only something that can be placed on a scale and measured in weight can be capable of producing a therapeutic effect. Homeopathy is a very powerful member of the family of energetic medicines.

Professor of Physics Cyril W. Smith from Salford University, Great Britain, who has conducted extensive research on applications of physics in biology and human health, asserts that homeopathic solutions are active energetic entities endowed with coherent and specific oscillations. He has stated that homeopathy cannot be explained by the limitations of chemistry. Instead, he says, *"physics and not chemistry is the science from which to seek explanations."* [13] Nobel Laureate in Physics of Cambridge University, Dr. Brian D. Josephson, and Professor of Aerospace Sciences and Dean Emeritus of the School of Engineering and Applied Science at Princeton University, Robert G. Jahn, are among the reputable scientists who agree with Professor Smith and do not see any flaws within scientific tenets of homeopathy as an energy-based medical system.

Q: How does the over-dilution of a crude chemical substance convert that substance into energy?

A: In order to answer this question, we need to consider some basic concepts which afford us a different angle from which to consider what the term "chemical substance" means. Whenever we refer to any substance or object in our environment, we perceive it causally and in a purely materialistic way that is limited by our five senses. This mode of perception prevents us from discerning much deeper underlying levels of Nature. There is another dimension to everything in Nature, including our environment and our bodies. This dimension—energy—is the deepest and the most fundamental of all. The various forms and interactions of energy comprise the main subject of the science of physics, which according to the National Science Education Standards, has been established as the most fundamental in the hierarchy of all sciences. In practical terms, "most fundamental" means that the laws and theories of physics must apply to other sciences and disciplines including chemistry, biology and medicine.

A branch of physics, quantum physics, studies the structure and composition of *atoms,* the building blocks of all substances or matter in the universe. Atoms are combined into larger structures—molecules—which in turn shape all matter, including the cells of Man.

Quantum physicists have discovered that atoms are themselves composed of about 60 different subatomic, or elementary, particles.

The process of homeopathic preparation is evidently capable of transferring energy and information from the subatomic domains of the original crude substance into homeopathic solutions. (For more details, refer to the Appendix at the end of this Chapter.)

Q: What proof is there that homeopathic preparations are indeed active energetic medicines?
A: Modern technologies using spectra-analysis obtained with the Raman-laser, infrared absorbance and nuclear magnetic resonance (NMR) have all confirmed the difference in emission patterns between homeopathic remedies and a placebo.[14–21] In addition, each homeopathic remedy was found to exhibit a unique NMR emission pattern.[22] Furthermore, substances that were both diluted and succussed to 30X potency according to full homeopathic method exhibited a specific band pattern in their emission spectra that was absent when the substances were merely diluted but not succussed.[23]

An international team of researchers, Prof. Cyril Smith of Great Britain and Dr. Christian Endler of Austria, obtained frequency measurements of homeopathic potencies. They determined, for example, that the homeopathic preparation of the thyroid hormone, thyroxine, in D5 potency, registered as 0.07 Hz. The frequency of the preparation continued to rise with each successive potentization cycle.[24]

The experiments of Physics Professor Wolfgang Ludwig of Germany recorded the specific electromagnetic frequencies emitted by several homeopathic remedies in support of this explanation. For example, a remedy of *Arnica* in 1000X or 1M potency gave off the frequency of 9.725 KHz.[25]

Professor G. Preparata, chairman of the Institute of Nuclear Physics in Milan, Italy, and his colleague, Professor Del Giudice, proposed a *superradiance theory* for homeopathic medicines whereby atoms of water and those of an original substance form stable, organized and energetically coherent units that emit characteristic energy patterns and resemble a network of mini-lasers.[26] These units are protected by hydrogen "shells" of water that enable the network to maintain a high degree of coherence by combating the natural propensity of any system toward increased disorder (*entropy*). The energy emitted by homeopathic preparations exerts its actions even through sealed glass vials. This was confirmed when the growth of animals exposed to sealed vials was accelerated.[27]

Stanford University Professor Emeritus of Materials Science, William A. Tiller, has explained that homeopathic preparations form two main energetic layers that become permanently imprinted into water media: one more superficial, primarily electric, and another, deeper and more subtle, mainly magnetic layer.[28]

While normal water has no net electrical charge, water containing IE clusters, found in homeopathic solutions, emits a small electric charge.[29]

Q: Even if homeopathic remedies contain some energy charge, why should it help heal the sick?
A: The reason homeopathic remedies are capable of producing therapeutic effects in the sick, is that humans are the ideal recipients of the energetic properties of homeopathic medicines. This is attributable largely to the energy fields of our cells that regulate our entire physiology, including our body chemistry. Even though research in this area began almost a century ago, it has only been with the development of more sophisticated research technology during the last several decades that this body of evidence has become convincing. These discoveries have enormous practical importance because they put energetic therapeutic interventions such as homeopathy on a firm scientific foundation. The brief account of this evidence presented here is intended to help the reader more fully appreciate the immense potential that homeopathy carries for chronic, acute and preventative medical care, especially in dealing with the effects of biological, toxicological or radioactive agents. In addition, this information will be very helpful to understanding the full advantage and superiority of both the energetic therapeutics and diagnostic methods based on this energy principle.

In the late 1800's, German chemist Baron von Reichenbach, famous for his discovery of creosote, claimed to have been able to imprint on photographic plates luminescent energetic rays radiating from human bodies, animals and plants.[30]

In 1923, Georges Lakhovsky, a Russian engineer working in France, built a simple apparatus capable of registering microvoltage measurements from human cells, plants and microbes. He was able to record the diverse oscillations in the radio and color frequency ranges emitted by living organisms. Studying human cells from a purely electrical engineering viewpoint, he found a striking similarity between the composition of a regular battery and that of a human cell. He described the ability of chromosomes and other cell structures composed of fat and protein to act as insulators and the ability of mineral-rich intracellular and extracellular fluids to generate electric charges. In his studies of normal and diseased cells, Lakhovsky found that there were marked differences in their oscillation patterns. Each group of cells emitted frequencies specific to its organ or tissue of origin. Cancerous cells emitted a different, abnormal pattern. Lakhovsky also discovered that harmful factors such as faulty nutrition, environmental pollutants containing toxic chemicals or heavy metals, bacteria or viruses weaken and distort cellular electro-magnetic fields prior to the onset of illness and death. After years of research and experimentation, he concluded that health is nothing but a state of electro-magnetic equilibrium of body cells, while diseases and death represent just the opposite—a broken energetic balance.

Quite prophetically, Lakhovsky surmised that health and disease represent an ongoing "war of radiations" between the body and harmful elements.[31] Based upon his theory that abnormal electromagnetic vibrations of cells play a primary role in the development of diseases, Lakhovsky built a radio-electrical apparatus which he called a "Multiple Wave Oscillator" to treat cancerous tumors. He conducted his experiments in the 1930's in various hospitals in Paris, treating many types of cancer, reportedly with good results. It was due to this success that the apparatus was used in 1937 in the treatment of Pope Pius XI, affording him a two-year remission from cancer. Some 50 years later, a Swedish radiologist, Prof. E.W. Nordenström of Sweden, has incorporated Lakhovsky's ideas into his successful treatment of terminal cancer patients.

In the 1920's, a Russian émigré and cell researcher working in Germany, cytologist Alexander Gurwitsch, photographed the energetic oscillations in the ultra-violet light spectrum emitted by plant cells during cell division in several well-conducted scientific experiments. Another European researcher, astronomer Albert Nodon of France, published his measurements of the electric charges emitted by human cells, insects and plants in October of 1927.[32] In 1930, Professor Guido Cremonese of Italy published a scientific monograph in which he displayed photographs of radiations from human blood and saliva using a special method that he devised.[33]

Another interesting phenomenon discovered by Gurwitsch was that these oscillations (or as they were called, "radiations") stimulated other living cells, even at distance. When a dividing onion root (a "sender") was separated by a sheet of quartz from a "receiver" (another onion root, yeast or bacteria), all of the "receivers" tested still demonstrated faster growth. In human tissues, Dr. Gurwitsch also found that the eye, blood and nerves were all emitters of radiations. Similar to the observations reported by other researchers, cancerous tissue radiated differently, with the blood of cancer patients demonstrating a poor radiance.[34,35]

Around the same time, Professor Harold Saxton Burr of Yale Medical School carried out his own investigation of human-energy related phenomena. His systematic measurements of the electromagnetic fields emitted by different body tissues and organs confirmed Lakhovsky's findings concerning the difference in the electrical emissions of healthy and diseased organs and tissues. Professor Burr concluded that these energetic fields control a primary function regulating all of our physiological and biochemical processes and may even constitute a blueprint for life itself (he named them "L-fields", with "L" representing Life).[36] These conclusions were echoed by George Crile, Sr., MD, the founder of the renowned Cleveland Clinic, who proclaimed that this area of medicine held unlimited potential for the future.[37]

Regretfully, the work of Burr and Crile ended with their deaths. American medicine, dominated and essentially controlled by the pharmaceutical industry, offered no inducements to spur research for energy medicine. Such interest might also have helped to establish credence in its main rival, homeopathy, and thus threatened the medical mainstream's market share and profits. Consequently, energy-related biomedical research received no funding. Nonetheless, scientists outside the United States continued to probe deeper into the energetic dimensions of Man.

In the early 1940's, a Hungarian-born biochemist and Nobel Laureate in Medicine, Albert Szent-Györgyï, discovered that proteins, the main components of cells and DNA, are capable of conducting electricity. He sharply criticized the prevailing medical establishment's obsession with solely biochemical and pharmaceutical processes and strongly recommended that energy be made an integral part of bio-medical research. Without this most essential energetic element, he warned, researchers were merely discovering more and more facts about "dead" tissues.

In 1979, British biophysicist P. E. Rapp presented a summary of 450 scientific experiments confirming that the energetic properties of cells play a crucial role in key physiological processes and functions in the living.[38]

Björn E.W. Nordenström, Professor of Radiology from Karolinska Institute in Sweden, described the whole array of electric components in and around human cells in his book, "Biologically Closed Electric Circuits."[39] Following Lakhovsky's path, he documented recoveries of far advanced terminal cancer patients who were treated with electrotherapy after conventional medicine failed. Supporting Nordenström's work, Soviet biophysicists identified the specific electromagnetic charges of the key cellular components, including the cell nucleus that contains chromosomes.[40]

Professor Robert Becker, MD, a pioneer of Electromedicine in the U.S. and Chief of Orthopedic Surgery at the VA Hospital of SUNY at Syracuse, was able to induce tissue and bone healing in many hopeless patients by applying small currents through the tissues' electrical pathways. Mainstream medicine, he said, was based upon a scientifically outdated model that relied exclusively on the chemical-pharmaceutical approach, to the exclusion of the more fundamental dimension of body energetics. As a result, he concluded, the tremendous healing potential of energy-based medicines such as homeopathy, acupuncture, visualization and electromedicine were neglected, to the great detriment of the public.

Many scientists in the USSR have probed deeply into the phenomenon of energy in the living. In the highly respected Kirov State University of Kazakhstan in Alma-Ata, near the Soviet Space Center, a group of biologists, biochemists and biophysicists undertook the study of energy in the living, using modern technology, including electron microscopy. In 1968, they announced that indeed all living things—plants, animals and humans—were endowed with both a purely physical body made of visible tissues and organs and its twin, an "energy body." They observed this body's motion through a powerful electron microscope. Based upon the appearance of this "energy body," they named it the *biological plasma body*. *Plasma* is a special type of physical matter, consisting of a highly charged state of subatomic particles, it is considered to be the fourth state of matter in addition to solids, liquids, and gases, and it can be quite chaotic. The scientists concluded that the living bioplasma appeared to possess a specific spatial organization unique to every organism, organ and tissue. Echoing Professor Burr's concept of *Life-fields,* they postulated that the biological plasma does indeed represent an organizing blueprint for the matrix of life. Furthermore, they theorized that the combined energy of plasma and atomic-molecular matter form the total energy reserve that is essential to all life, and confirmed Dr. Hahnemann's assertion of a crucial role of body energy or *vital force* (the main target of homeopathic medicines) in healing. The scientists observed that exposure to toxic substances or stressful emotional stimuli changed the cellular energy emission patterns from normal to pathological.

Their work underscored the importance of therapies, such as homeopathy, that act at an energy level. With the advancement of scientific research technology, the number of discoveries concerning the human energy field mushroomed. For example, in 1967 a magnetic field around the human heart was observed with a sophisticated Superconducting Quantum Interference Device *(SQUID)* at the Massachusetts Institute of Technology in Cambridge, Massachusetts. Three years later, observations of the human brain offered evidence that the magnetic field extended beyond the boundaries of the head itself.[41] Since the early 1980's, Magnetic Resonance Imaging (MRI) has become commonplace in Western medicine. Interestingly enough, MRI is based upon its capacity to record innate magnetic properties of human cells. Professor Tiller believes that the magnetic elements in living cells are repositories for voluminous amounts of information, the pathological content of which contributes to the development and sustainment of chronic diseases.[42,43] All of the major assaults (toxic pollutants, infectious agents, or physical and emotional traumas) that the body is not able to overcome become imprinted onto these cellular recordings in a

CD-like fashion, and then continuously feed back into the body's chemistry, altering it adversely. This "cellular memory" could explain the tenacity of chronic diseases and the inability of conventional pharmaceutical methods to eradicate them. Drugs which act through chemistry, the most superficial level of Man's physiology, simply cannot erase pathological information residing within our cells. Professor Tiller and other researchers attribute the memory-retaining functions of the body to the previously described magnetic elements of water. The last constitutes a major part of our cells.

In 1994, two biophysicists from the Max-Planck Institute of Physics in Gottingen, Germany, Drs. Erwin Neher and Bert Sackmann, were awarded a Nobel Prize for their discovery of the essential role that the flow of charged atoms—the *ions* of body fluids and tissues—play in physiological processes in living cells. Similarly, German physicist Professor Herbert Fröhlich of the University of Liverpool, a world-recognized authority on human energy research, summarized his 50 years of research in the field by concluding that every structure in the body, including the entire chemistry of the body, down to the chromosomes, is energy-operated and driven by electromagnetic fields that are created by flows of charged ions.[44] He received the Max Planck Medal, the highest award for physics in Germany. Along with his countryman, Professor Fritz-Albert Popp, Professor Fröhlich established that cells in the body interact through coherent oscillations. In health, these oscillations are robust and precise. They can be likened to miniature radio stations, exchanging clear and synchronized signals.

If one considers that every human cell contains 100,000 genes and chemistry of a single cell is run by about 3,000 enzymes, and that Man's body on a whole contains some 75 trillion cells, with as many as 100,000 chemical reactions taking place in each cell every second, it would be impossible for the body to maintain such enormous biochemical machinery or to adapt it quickly to ongoing stresses by relying on the relatively slow speed of chemical reactions.[45,46] Professors Fröhlich and Popp have demonstrated that electromagnetic communication between cells constitutes the primary process governing chemical reactions. Professor Cyril W. Smith, in particular, emphasized that living systems make much more precise use of physics than most man-made machines.[47,48]

The existence of an electromagnetic charge across the outer level of every living cell, the cell membrane, has been known for a long time. The cell membrane contains very specialized structures, called receptors, whose main function is to recognize the key components of our body chemistry: hormones, enzymes, neurotransmitters, immune system modulators and other elements. These membrane-bound receptors are the main gatekeepers of our cellular chemistry. Most drug research is based upon receptor functions. In addition to their chemical functions, receptors also possess an electromagnetic charge and can be influenced effectively via delivery of even small electromagnetic signals of a magnitude similar to those contained within homeopathic remedies. For example, a homeopathic remedy, *Chelidonium,* affects liver cholesterol receptors and reduces serum total cholesterol concentration. Unlike cholesterol-lowering drugs, it is free of dangerous side-effects.[49]

Even DNA itself has been found to oscillate in resonance with frequencies in the microwave range and is capable of responding to electromagnetic frequencies.[50,51] Professor Popp demonstrated that DNA performs its regulatory functions and receives feedback information from chemical reactions via tiny electromagnetic charges—photons.[52] Furthermore, Soviet researchers found that even after DNA molecules were physically removed from a solution, residual oscillations of these molecules remained present, which they called "phantom DNA."[53]

California physicist Dr. William Adey of Loma Linda University School of Medicine also concluded that the most fundamental mechanism of communication between cells occurs through weak electromagnetic signals. These lead to the binding of hormones, neurotransmitters or antibodies of the immune system and other important biochemical elements to receptors precisely where they are required—at their expected action sites.[54] Professor Del Giudice proposed a concept of "intelligent biochemistry" whereby our entire body chemistry and physiology operate through distinct energetic codes, signals and frequencies.[55,56] He also agreed with the theory that homeostasis in humans is maintained through a widespread network of cellular and molecular mini-radio stations, which act as transmitters and receivers, communicating with one another within corresponding frequency ranges.[57–59] Research performed in the

USSR confirmed that living cells do not even need to be in physical contact for chemical reactions to occur. In a very interesting experiment, scientists placed two identical and healthy live cell cultures in adjacent, but hermetically sealed containers separated by a quartz barrier permeable to the ultraviolet radiations emitted by the cell cultures. Then they introduced a lethal virus into one of the cultures. Surprisingly, the cell culture that was not directly contaminated also died. When the experiment was repeated, this time with the quartz barrier replaced with an ordinary glass, also impermeable to ultraviolet radiation, the culture with the introduced virus perished but the other remained healthy. Similar results were obtained when the experiment was repeated with a variety of toxic agents.[60]

In a series of experiments conducted in medical facilities in London and Dallas, Texas, allergic patients displayed exactly the same allergic reactions whether exposed to the actual chemical allergens or to certain electromagnetic frequencies.[61-65] The researchers also discovered that the patients emitted electromagnetic radiations in the course of their allergy attacks. Conversely, allergic attacks could be neutralized by either exposing the subjects to certain electromagnetic frequencies or by having the subjects drink water that had been exposed to these frequencies. Water, as already mentioned, is an ideal repository for information essential to homeopathic action.

In a review of the literature, 81 scientific research studies concerning the physiologic role of photon emission in the regulation of various aspects of cellular metabolism in the living were scrutinized by scientists from the Department of Molecular Cell Biology of University of Utrecht, Netherlands. The review confirmed the important role of electromagnetic communication in cell functioning.[66]

This vast body of scientific evidence makes it apparent that the physiology of all living systems is being run via computer-like electromagnetic communications. Furthermore, homeopathic remedies, which contain stored diverse and specific energetic information, may be able to interact with the endogenous energetic communication system in the living and provide stimulating and correcting signals that promote self-repair and healing. Homeopathy is indeed unique among all therapies in its ability to influence cellular memory.

Q: How do remedies made out of all kinds of poisons (toxic plants, metals, snake or spider venoms) therapeutically "match" a person in the first place?

A: The very existence of an illness automatically implies a lack of proper physiological adaptation—i.e., the body has failed to overcome the factors that have fostered disease and therefore needs help in raising adaptive capacity. There are several reasons why seemingly foreign and even poisonous substances can restore failed adaptation. One of them is the fact that the human body contains virtually all the elements in the Periodic Table, including metals, minerals, trace and radioactive elements, gases, and others. All of these elements, in single or combined forms, are also contained in all other living beings or organic substance. They form the key ingredients of cellular structures, proteins, fats, and sugars, among other components. Inorganic elements, such as minerals, metals, and trace elements exert a significant effect on the metabolism of protein, fat, and sugar in humans by complementing the thousands of enzymes that regulate metabolism. Thus the molecules and atoms in a "poison" are also found in a human body; neither is composed of components alien to the other. Thus, properly determined and administered, the elements can be "matched."

Correlatively, homeopathic substances can trigger restoration of adaptation ability because at the subatomic level, every living or inorganic substance is composed of the same elementary particles which form atomic energy fields.

Another even more subtle aspect concerning elementary particles is that they all had the same place of origin. Whether one subscribes to the Big-Bang theory or the theory of Divine Creation, subatomic particles came into existence at some point from the same place of origin. Since that distant time, both the subatomic particles and the living or inorganic systems that they formed, have undergone countless processes to adapt to their corresponding environments—some on the surface of the Earth, some within the depth of its soil, some on the peaks of frigid, windy mountains, some in the oceans, others in the burning heat of desert sands, or in the damp and rainy jungles. Even poisonous or toxic properties of some substances resulted from some type of adaptational or formative processes. According to quantum physics, these adaptational processes have not merely been left in the past, but have been ingrained and recorded as the information memory fields of subatomic energy domains. This information, applied to medicines, can be of great benefit to humans in their adaptational struggle against whatever factors cause illness.

Perhaps this is why, as an example, a homeopathic remedy made out of the plant *Aconite (Aconitum napellus),* which grows on mountain and hilltops, is indispensable for a person who experiences a sudden and violent cold after being exposed to cold air or a draft of wind. This exposure resembles the natural habitat of the plant, which often is exposed to sudden cold winds. Many heart patients experiencing bad angina report that this remedy works better than any heart medications on cold winter days. As an extra benefit, homeopathic remedies work not only by relieving their sufferers of discomforting symptoms in the short-term, but also, as a rule, lead to long-lasting resistance against corresponding pernicious factors. In contrast, pharmaceutical agents must be taken repeatedly and merely suppress symptoms under adverse circumstances. They are unable to induce either true healing or adaptation.

Similarly, *Dulcamara (Solanium dulcamara)* grows in damp and shady places. Its thin branches have a propensity to grow and entwine around any available support. The homeopathic remedy made out of this plant, *Dulcamara,* is very effective for a person who is maladapted to humidity and who needs to move physically in order to improve his chronic arthritic pains.

Sepia officinalis, the cuttlefish of the mollusk family, resembles in shape a human uterus. Over the last two hundred years, the homeopathic remedy *Sepia,* made from the ink sack of the cuttlefish, has been a savior to women all over the world suffering from a long list of gynecological and hormonal problems when *Sepia* matched their symptoms. Perhaps the similarities in the shape are coincidental. Perhaps there are deeper phenomena of Nature in play whose workings we have yet to grasp.

A strictly individualized use, or a "match" of a classical homeopathic prescription is based upon a careful analysis of multiple features of an ill person and those of a remedy known to provide energetic correction in these circumstances.

Whether homeopathic remedies prescribed are based upon this kind of a "match" or upon the knowledge of exact offending biological, chemical or nuclear agents, the *gating theory* of molecular biology sheds further light on their mechanism of action.[67] This concept, in a nutshell, implies that our cells can respond to and process only so much information at one time. From this perspective, if a homeopathic remedy such as anthrax or a sleep gas engages the cells in a communication process, the result will be a partial or complete cellular disengagement from the pathological connection with the corresponding disease producing agent(s). This mechanism leads to a better understanding of the seemingly irrational "law of similars" or one of "the same." The more specific the homeopathic energetic print-outs of the actual offending agents or disease process on the whole can be, the more capable they are of engaging the cells at the action sites of that agent or disease process inside a body and cutting off their corresponding actions.

Fractal geometry, a recent development in mathematics and computer science, may enhance our understanding of the subtle energetic nature of homeopathic remedies.[68] This new discipline has established that most things in Nature, including human cells, contain geometrical patterns—*fractals*—that repeat themselves on both the microscopic and macroscopic levels of structure.[69,70] These fractal patterns also exist in atoms and are formed by subatomic particles.[71] The famous French mathematician of the 19th century, Joseph Fourrier, established a formula (the *Fourrier transform*) whereby, through a set of mathematical equations, it is possible to translate geometrical wave forms into their energy equivalents. One contemporary hypothesis states that the preparation process of a homeopathic remedy propels an element of information gain as the fractal patterns in the solution gain in precision with each successive dilution and succussion. All of this data further supports the notion that the efficacy of homeopathic remedies lies in the delivery of very specific information as energetic signals.[71a] These signals are needed by the body to increase its adaptation capacity, in order to progress from a state of disorder and disease toward a state of order and health. An interconnectedness and a potential for therapeutic symbiosis among all things in Nature exists on a deep energetic level. Homeopathy has found a method of tapping into this symbiotic pool of Nature to bring about therapeutic regulation and healing.

Because the proper choice of energetic therapeutic signals is all-important, the purely chemical content of an original source becomes irrelevant. All that counts is the proper choice, timing and intensity of a signal, i.e. its potency. Moreover, as recent advancements in computer science, mathematics and physics have demonstrated, humans appear to respond ideally to such signals because their physiologic functions sustain continuous wave-like oscillations fluctuating between energetic order and disorder *(chaos)*.[72] It has been demonstrated that the activity of our enzymes, hormones, organs, heart and brain rhythms constantly vary according to these dynamic fluctuating patterns.[73–76] Because we humans are open living systems, we are constantly subjected to many incoming messages or inputs of diverse nature: emotional, nutritional, atmospherical, toxicological and biological. Therefore, we cannot maintain our physiology in a fixed state because it must oscillate constantly in response to these inputs. In health, these fluctuations tend to remain closer to order than to chaos. Under the impact of adverse inputs, a given body function or system begins to move toward disorder and, if not redirected, approaches a point of *bifurcation* (i.e., a "fork in the road"). This reflects a condition of a precarious energetic state where the affected system or function becomes increasingly likely to lose its state of normalcy and transform into a state of pathology.

It has been determined that while at a bifurcation point, a system will become increasingly sensitive to even the weakest oscillatory signals. If that signal has a special meaning for a system's needs at the time, the system will respond with movement back toward order.[77] In a way, the body resembles a tightrope walker suspended between two towers. When he stands firmly with both feet on one of the towers, even a strong wind does not affect him. Yet once he steps on the rope and continues his precarious walk, even the slightest motion of air can make him lose his balance or help him to regain stability.

"The Butterfly Effect" offers a now-classic example of a weak signal that can produce major change within even a large fluctuating system. It has been established through computer-generated mathematical models that under certain conditions, the flap of a butterfly's wings in Brazil may set off or abort a tornado in Texas.[78] By taking simultaneous advantage of the instability of systems in disorder and their enhanced sensitiveness to corrective signals, the properly prescribed homeopathic medicines are capable of playing a major role in empowering living systems to regain states of health and increased order.

Appendix to Chapter 1

Electrons are the most abundant subatomic particles. Although electrons are not the smallest of these particles, they are infinitesimally small—one electron has a mass of only ~9.10×10^{-31}kg.

Electrons are known to possess electrical charge and because of their perpetual motion emit waves that represent electromagnetic energy. The *photons,* massless wave-particles, represent the smallest unit—quanta—of electromagnetic energy. Because the waves travel at the extreme velocity of the speed of light, they form very powerful force-fields.

Each substance in the universe has its own number of subatomic particles within atoms positioned in specific configurations in relation to each other. These two characteristics of subatomic particles, their number and positions, generate an energetic field for each substance that determines its identity and its material and chemical properties. In essence, this field represents the "energetic passport-ID" of each substance. These fields also determine the chemical reactions and physical interactions between substances, including the chemical and physiologic processes that take place within our bodies. Consequently, subatomic energy fields shape all chemistry, including our own body chemistry. This part of quantum physics was named Quantum Electrodynamics and several Nobel prizes in physics were awarded for its discovery.[79,80]

Less than 1% of the total space within atoms is filled with relatively solid matter—the *nucleus*—which consists of heavier subatomic particles—*protons* and *neutrons*. The weights of the other subatomic particles are so negligible that they are considered to be practically massless. This means that practically 99% of the atomic space is composed of force-fields of subatomic particles and not the particles themselves. In a purely materialistic sense, atoms are largely energy-filled empty space. Yet these force-fields are so powerful that even the apparently hardest, most solid and densest materials, such as stainless steel, rock, or concrete, contain more empty space than physical matter. The marble floor that we walk on, the hardiest military machines, and other structures that appear to be extremely dense, are all mostly empty space. The reason we do not fall through the marble floor when we walk on it, or that tanks and bomb shelters are able to sustain powerful rocket impacts, is because of the strength of the force-fields being generated constantly between the subatomic particles.

Indeed, one of the cornerstones of modern physics, Einstein's Theory of Relativity, states that these force-fields constitute the very essence of all matter in Nature. The Theory of Relativity emphasizes the dual nature of all matter: Energy fields and physical matter are manifestations of the same thing. According to Einstein, the energy-field is dominant; it constitutes "the only true reality" because physical matter represents only an extended form of energy. We refer in our daily life to any object or substance as a physical entity simply because we are not accustomed to think of an "energy field" of gold, asbestos, anthrax, smallpox or car, although strictly speaking, it would be more correct scientifically. We do, however, harness the power of the energy fields of subatomic particles in the generation of the two main energy sources for our industrial and technological development—electricity and magnetism.

Another example of the immense power contained within the unseen microworld of atoms is a domain called *vacuum*. In our common understanding, vacuum usually is associated with a space that is deemed to be empty or devoid of anything. Yet a vacuum is a region where the density of bound energy is the highest and the most abundant that exists within the known universe. According to Professor William A. Tiller, the energy density of a vacuum is so immense that the total intrinsic energy contained within one single hydrogen atom is about one trillion times larger than that contained in the physical mass of all the planets plus all the stars in the entire known cosmos out to a radius of 20 billion light years.[81] The vacuum gives birth to subatomic particles and is known to interact with them to some degree. The enormous energy forces that are being released from atoms and which produce the monstrous destructive power of nuclear weapons are only feeble examples of the immense potential energy harbored within the subatomic world. This invisible microworld provides the powerful energetic essence of homeopathic remedies.

During the preparation of a homeopathic remedy, a number of mechanisms are involved in producing an energetic medicine. Their complete explanation requires a detailed account of the laws and principles of quantum physics, quantum chemistry, crystallography and other scientific disciplines. This is beyond the scope of this book. Nonetheless, we can grasp the basic processes that convert an "over-diluted substance" into a homeopathic remedy.

Assume we begin with a colony of anthrax bacteria suspended in a solution that we intend to turn into a homeopathic remedy. As we proceed with the homeopathic preparation process, we withdraw one drop of this solution and place it in a ½ oz. glass bottle that contains 99 drops of water. We then succuss this bottle ten times mechanically. What happens during this succussion process to the atoms of the anthrax bacteria? Their subatomic particles receive an extra energy boost from the *kinetic energy* of the motion produced by the agitation. This is the same form of energy that transforms falling water into electricity at hydroelectric power stations. Each time we agitate the bottle, the energy level of the subatomic particles escalates to a more excited state. This change affects not only the particles themselves but also their energy waves and force-fields. According to the findings of quantum physics, every time we raise the energy of each sequential dilution we preserve and enhance the information contained in the solution's force-fields.

As we proceed further with the serial dilution process we also continue mechanical succussion, simultaneously increasing both the dilution and the energy level of the subatomic particles of the anthrax bacteria. Quantum physics also predicts that gains in excitation and energy significantly increase the life spans of such particles; they become longer-lived *quasi-particles,* able to establish more stable fields of information within the homeopathic anthrax solution. The mechanical impacts of succussion may also increase the solution's photon emission off orbital electrons, thereby conveying the energetic information that pertained to the original substance.

In summary, during homeopathic preparation the concentration of material substance and the energetic charge contained within the solution proceed in opposite directions. The substance's energy charge continues to increase as the quantity progressively diminishes.

A second aspect of homeopathic energetic pharmaco-dynamics involves the properties of water. Water contains electric currents and generates electromagnetic waves.[82] Extensive research has established that combined and repetitive dilution and succussion allows the formation of highly organized global networks of clusters of water molecules. Resembling crystals, these clusters are capable of retaining the information within the original solutions. Named I_E *clusters* by scientists at the California Institute of Technology, they can be thought of as microscopic ice crystals within water media.[83–85]

The properties of I_E *clusters* allow the transfer of data contained within clusters long after the last molecule of the original substance has been removed from the solution. The I_E *clusters* in such homeopathic solutions are able to interact with one another via resonance communication in a manner similar to the way radio transmitters interact as they emit electromagnetic vibrations and reflect signals to one another. This confers increased stability and a coherent information pattern on the entire communication network throughout the newly formed solution. The form and vibration pattern of I_E *clusters* are specific for each given substance. The discovery of I_E *clusters* within water and their peculiar properties of data replication and storage with subsequent cycles of dilution and succussion has added further to the understanding of the homeopathic method of preparation. Their existence provides one premise for homeopathic remedies being energetic medicines, which retain their specific information over the long-term.

Chapter 2

What is Hormesis, its Relationship to Homeopathy and Why is it Being Silenced?

Additional evidence in support of the scientific validity of homeopathy comes from the science of toxicology, which studies the effects of toxic substances on humans. For nearly a century, toxicologists have known of a very strange phenomenon called *hormesis.* This term describes the paradoxical behavior of very diluted amounts of toxic agents. When ingested in homeopathic-like doses, such agents can offer health benefits. This phenomenon reaffirms the tenet put forward by the famous Swiss Professor, Theophrastus Paracelsus, MD. As long ago as in 1567, Paracelsus declared that, strictly speaking, there were no poisons or medications in medicine—it was the *dose* that determined whether a substance could cause harm or heal. Paracelsus has been considered a medical genius and an exceptionally gifted healer by many familiar with his work. He was the first to correctly predict the existence of germs. He incorporated principles of mind-body medicine in his medical practice, and administered low doses of toxic metals, infected body fluids, and other noxious substances with great success.[86]

Hormesis has been formalized by what is known in pharmacology as the *Arndt-Schultz Law* and *Hueppe's Rule:* High doses kill; medium doses harm, and low doses benefit. Mainstream toxicologists and pharmacologists maintain that low doses have no effect and are useless, yet extensive evidence leaves no doubt that hormesis is a real, natural phenomenon.

Thanks to the knowledge of its existence—we are compelled to accept, seemingly at odds with our culturally-conditioned understanding, a whole array of evidence and observations, among them: that 100,000 victims of the nuclear bombing of Hiroshima and Nagasaki enjoyed a longer survival than their counterparts who were exposed to lower amounts of radiation; that certain ranges of electromagnetic radiation produce beneficial effects on human cells; that immune stimulants may suppress or enhance cancer growth or immunity depending on the dose; that a powerful carcinogen, when fed in low doses to 24,000 animals, protected them against cancer; and that in contrast, hospital and pharmacy personnel who handled anti-cancer chemotherapy drugs developed more cancers.[87]

Over the years, stimulatory and overall beneficial effects have been observed in response to the following agents when administered in highly diluted solutions: *Metals:* arsenic, cadmium, chromium, cobalt, copper, lead, lithium, manganese, mercury, platinum, silver, thallium, thorium; *Metallic Compounds:* barium, nickel, strontium, tin, zinc; Chemicals: benzene, cyanide, chlorobiphenyls, toluene, xylene, phenol, crude oil, DDT, malathione, pesticides, toxic gas of carbon tetrachloride; *Carcinogenic Chemical Compounds:* 3,4-benzpyrene, 1,2,5,6-dibenzanthracene and 3-methylcholanthrene. Small doses of *ionizing radiation* and *antibiotics* promote rather than suppress bacteria growth. In several large human studies, low-dose exposure to the radioactive elements plutonium, radium, and radon was found to reduce cancer incidence. Small amounts of lead have stimulated nerve cell growth. The homeopathic remedy, *Plumbum metallicum* (potentized lead), has become known for its effectiveness in the treatment of neurologic conditions.[88–116]

University of Connecticut pharmacologist Patricia J. Neafsey summarized, in her essay, *Longevity Hormesis, A Review,* the beneficial effects of hormesis on animals, citing over 100 scientific references. She emphasized the abundant positive effects of low doses of toxic substances, including enhanced functioning of the liver cytochrome P-450 enzyme system, the key detoxifying system in mammals; improved viability in terms of growth, weight gain, development, reproductive life span, and wound healing; resistance to infection, radiation damage, cancer, and diseases in general; and, not least, a longer life span.[117]

One of the most recent confirmations of a hormetic homeopathic phenomenon was demonstrated in experiments involving T-lymphocytes, the key elements of our immune system. T-lymphocytes that were subjected to high concentrations of antigens died, while low doses of the same antigens stimulated the autoreactivity of these cells.[118,119] These and similar findings support the scientific plausibility of homeopathy as "applied hormesis."[120,121]

Despite the formulation of the Arndt-Schultz Law, how low doses of toxic agents induce beneficial responses is not fully understood. One hypothesis is that the body naturally resists foreign substances such as toxins and drugs. This hypothesis is consistent with *Le Chatelier's Principle,* which states that when a force is imposed upon a system, it reacts to nullify the effect of that force. Whereas high doses may overwhelm the system, minute doses of toxins serve to irritate and stimulate the defense mechanisms, boosting immune and metabolic capacity to a level which benefits the system as a whole. These benefits are manifested as increased growth and improved overall health.[122] The dose deemed necessary has been termed the *sufficient challenge* and is very similar in concept to the miniscule doses of allergens employed by allergists to challenge and raise the body's defense against allergenic agents. Likewise, a study published in August 2002 in *The New England Journal of Medicine* reported the significant benefits of the diluted form of a known neurotoxin—botulism—when administered to neurological patients.

Researcher and toxicologist, H. F. Smyth, Jr., in his review article, *Sufficient Challenge,* pointed out that a dose-related response to a low dose of a harmful substance parallels well-accepted principles of the response to stress.[123] A cornerstone law of physiology of living organisms, for which Austrian-born endocrinologist Hans Selye was awarded a Nobel Prize in medicine, states that the body mounts a maximum response to stress at its onset but as the stress continues and reaches a high level, adaptational mechanisms become exhausted and fail. Smyth emphasized that homeopathy is the only medical system that puts the concept of *sufficient challenge to widespread use:* "Here a trace of a chemical is relied upon to cure an injury such as would be caused by a lot of the chemical—a hair of the dog which bit you."

Even though hormesis cannot be denied, it has not been embraced by mainstream toxicologists, who have chosen to study harmful, not beneficial, effects of poisons.

There has always been a tendency among the majority of modern scientists to stay within the established consensus of what constitutes "perfect knowledge", according to a given stage of "accepted knowledge" and within the mainstream of "organized science." Ironically, however, as pointed out by pharmacologist Dr. D. Steinbach, "It is incontrovertible fact that our state of knowledge at any given time also reveals our state of ignorance."[124,125]

Thomas Kuhn, an internationally known science analyst and philosopher, has described the pressure exerted within the field. According to Kuhn, "accepted knowledge" defines "normal science" for fear that disputing "accepted knowledge" may upset the establishment to the detriment of one's career.

Indeed, Kuhn states that new ideas are not necessarily required or encouraged. Quite the opposite; discoveries that threaten established theories are resented and sometimes suppressed.[126]

This is especially true among scientists who depend heavily on Federal research grants and pharmaceutical company research contracts. Obviously, drug companies are interested primarily, if not exclusively, in pharmaceutical patents and their own financial prosperity, even if these come into sharp conflict with "perfect knowledge." The Federal bodies that distribute research funding are staffed solely with mainstream "normal scientists." It should not be surprising that if these "normal scientists" do not agree that hormesis and homeopathy are part of "accepted knowledge," they will not fund such research. On the other hand, if "normal scientists" believe that dietary fat is bad and that the American people should gorge themselves with carbohydrates, funding to support this dubious view is abundantly available. Indeed, the astronomical amount of $500 million has been wasted in tenacious and yet repeatedly unsuccessful attempts to demonstrate the superiority of dietary sugars. The end result has been tremendous harm to the health of the entire population.[127]

Raymond Damadian, the engineer who invented the indigenous energetic imaging technique, Magnetic Resonance Imaging (MRI), has written a bitter account of his long struggle to obtain funding from the medical establishment for his research. Mr. Damadian reports that mainstream scientists simply said, "we don't believe in it." When funds for his work ran out, he literally passed a hat around in an Armenian church, and even tried to appeal to then-President-elect Jimmy Carter for help by making a pilgrimage to his brother

Billy's bar. Brother Billy, however, was unable to relate to the subject matter and threw him out.[128]

This bias against alternative medical concepts and approaches has been documented by a study sponsored by the National Academy of Sciences. The Academy scrutinized the peer review system, and concluded that an endorsement or rejection had very little to do with the scientific merit of presented ideas, but rather, with whether the reviewers were sympathetic or hostile to the hypothesis in question. These findings were suppressed for several years.[129]

Perhaps it should not be surprising, then, that one of the pioneers of U.S. electromedicine, Professor Robert O. Becker, M.D, two-time nominee for the Nobel Prize in Medicine, should find his lab equipment and records dumped one day on the sidewalk outside the university hospital where he was conducting his research.[130]

Despite the numerous well-designed research studies documenting the effectiveness of hormesis, the sobering social reality is that it remains as much an orphan in toxicology as homeopathy does within conventional medicine. As much as homeopathic remedies' infinitesimal concentrations and energy-based therapeutics puzzle "normal scientists" and shatter the mainstream pharmaceutical paradigm, the hormetic effects of low doses of poisons challenge the long-established platform of mainstream toxicology that poisons kill in high doses or do nothing in low doses.

Edward Calabrese, internationally recognized Professor of Toxicology at the University of Massachusetts at Amherst, has presented several major disincentives for individual toxicologists to pursue the advancement of hormesis:

- *Ideological bias* against finding that substances previously considered to be toxic may cause beneficial responses
- *Scarcity of funding* for high-volume studies
- *Mainstream training*—toxicological education exclusively emphasizes high-dose end-point responses; assessments of therapeutic benefits lies beyond the scope of typical toxicological study and objectives
- *Federal grants are a risky proposition*—the likelihood that grant proposals for hormesis-related research will be rejected is very high; many researchers depend on grants for their salaries[131]

But the greatest roadblock to the study of hormesis is, of course, its close resemblance to the principles of homeopathy. According to Professor Calabrese, hormesis is, thus, is deemed "guilty by association."[132]

In her book, *The Dose Makes the Poison,* toxicologist M. Alice Ottoboni underscores the persistence with which toxicologists shy away from acknowledging hormesis, even though *"every toxicologist involved in research with toxic chemical exposure is well aware of its existence. The phenomenon of beneficial effects from trace exposures to foreign chemicals, although often a subject of conversation among toxicologists . . . is rarely mentioned in the scientific literature."*[133] Even when research results clearly confirm hormetic effects, they are not mentioned directly in the "abstracts" where results are summarized. To save time, the abstract is usually all that is screened by the media or even many scientists themselves. *"It is only by careful perusal of the data tables and figures presented in the body of the text that the phenomenon is revealed. Such subtleties are lost on people who read only the abstracts of scientific papers."*

In a review article dedicated to hormesis, *"The Occurrence of Chemically Induced Hormesis,"* the authors reported that regretfully neither the term *hormesis* nor its related key word names—*hormoligosis, Arndt-Schultz Law,* or *sufficient challenge*—were mentioned in some of the major information retrieval systems concerning chemistry, medicine, or science in general.[134]

Another group of researchers from three university centers in Germany reported that they had encountered the same information blackout when they set out to gather all the available data on the subject of hormesis; it could not be accessed through any of the major medical, toxicological and science-related search engines.[135]

It should come as no surprise that studies conducted with homeopathic remedies that demonstrate the successful detoxification or health benefits have been dismissed by the "normal science" press. The main reason for this information blackout is that the majority of medical peer-reviewed journals, those preferentially entered into search engines, are reluctant to accept for publication studies concerning homeopathy or alternative medicine in general. The formal reason often given is that such studies "are not conducted well enough." Certainly when a common bias exists, the interpretation of the data of any study can be and is a very subjective process. Such studies are scrutinized excessively and often the end result is that most of the time no homeopathy research is deemed to be "good enough." Notably, a group of non-homeopath researchers from Great Britain concluded: *"Many homeopathic trials with positive results are accepted for publication only by so-called 'alternative' journals with limited exposure, where those with more negative results are likely to be published by orthodox journals, leading to reinforcement of the ideas already held by readers of these journals. Those members of the scientific community who are interested in homeopathic research often find accessibility to homeopathic journals difficult."*[136] Also, several good books that contain serious scientific analysis of homeopathy are in very limited circulation in English and, therefore, are costly and do not enjoy a wide public or professional exposure.

It is not surprising that in the environment where homeopathy has been turned into a sort of "stealth medicine," media coverage is laden with gross misrepresentations and outright misinformation that only reaffirms general misconceptions concerning this very powerful medical system. "Investigative reporters" who set out on a speedy "quack buster" mission to crucify homeopathy are usually too lazy to work through the laborious process of obtaining and scrutinizing the scientific literature. Instead, they resort to obtaining the opinions of conventional medical specialists associated with acclaimed medical schools and with "good credentials" to add the necessary "beef" to their opinions. The travesty of this kind of public education lies in the fact that the specialists are as ignorant about homeopathy (and most other subjects concerning alternative medicine) as the reporter. The problem is that a reporter often is not aware of the educational limitations of the experts and engages the specialists in a proverbial "blind leading the blind" interview. Without having to be concerned that the learned men will somehow ruin his mission of nailing these "quack homeopaths," the "truth seeker" feeds them naïve and biased questions concerning homeopathy, and the learned men simply confirm the reporter's biases.

An example of this "educational" approach was published in the famous consumer-oriented periodical, *Consumer Reports.*[137] In this "journalistic opus," the reporter attacked homeopathy on the basis that the high dilutions of high potency homeopathic remedies have lost all of the original substance. While neglecting to account for homeopathic action based on the laws of quantum physics rather than traditional chemistry, he avoided confronting the strengths of homeopathy. Even though the article included the cliché that homeopathy violates the laws of physics and biology, the report failed to substantiate this or quote a single physicist who could articulate these alleged "violations." The general consensus of the experts concerning homeopathic remedies was that "almost certainly, it's a placebo treatment."

Regretfully, this interview on the whole expresses the biased and ignorant attitude toward alternative medicine held by many of the mainstream "public educators" of high academic stature within allopathic medicine. These attitudes are widely publicized through the various media and are given the appearance of *bona fide* medical knowledge. Unfortunately, the public, at large, is unable to scrutinize scientific statements, and is easily misled by these recommendations. As a result, it is often denied far superior therapeutic options for themselves and their families.[138] (For details concerning general understanding of scientific process, refer to the Appendix following this chapter.) The practice of accepting a statement on faith merely because it is uttered by experts who are "supposed to know better" has been characterized by the former MIT scholar Gerald Schroeder, PhD: "It is hard not to be fooled by foolish arguments when they originate from intelligent foolers."[139]

One of the *Consumer Reports'* experts was a skeptical psychiatrist from a reputable New York hospital. In contrast, however, psychiatrist Jonathan R.T. Davidson, MD of Duke University, has utilized homeopathy successfully over many years in the treatment of a number of mental health problems, and takes the opposite position. Dr. Davidson has asserted that in addition to their effectiveness, homeopathic remedies are free of the "unacceptable side effects, hazardous interactions and dangerous overdoses" which are all too common when psychotropic drugs are administered.[140]

Homeopathy vs. Conventional Medicine—More Questions and Answers

Q: Theoretical science is all well and good, but is there any scientific evidence that homeopathy works?

A: Yes, such evidence does exist. In 1991 the *British Medical Journal* published a review article in which the investigators analyzed the results of 107 controlled clinical trials of the safety and effectiveness of homeopathic remedies. The investigators concluded that nearly 80% of these controlled clinical trials, considered to provide the best evidence of the effectiveness of a medical treatment, were of sufficiently high quality to demonstrate the effectiveness of homeopathic remedies.[141] In 1997, another major British medical journal, *The Lancet,* published a larger review of the results of 186 clinical trials of homeopathic remedies. The analysis was performed by several prestigious universities in Germany and the United States, including the U.S. National Institutes of Health (NIH). Despite the investigators' doubts concerning the scientific plausibility of homeopathy, they concluded that homeopathic remedies were intrinsically active and not merely placebo treatments.[142]

Q: If homeopathy is based on so much solid scientific evidence, why does it appear to be in such conflict with conventional medicine?

A: There is never a conflict between sciences; there only are conflicts between the people who work within science, the scientists themselves. By definition, the very essence of science is to study Nature and to understand her workings and laws. These workings and laws cannot be in competition. They can only complement one another. An American physicist, Nobel Prize Laureate Professor Murray Gell-Mann, described Nature as a multi-level structure and stated that the purpose of science is to investigate the laws of every level "from the top down and from the bottom up in order to build staircases between them."[143]

Every science or discipline *chooses* to study and explore its own level within this structure and to share observations and experimental results. These findings may be discoveries, new theories, or even breakthroughs. Yet, it must be remembered that scientists *choose* to study a certain level of Nature within a framework, or *paradigm,* bounded by the theories and assumptions of that particular worldview. Consequently, their understanding of findings, discoveries, and breakthroughs is limited by the framework within which they work and think. That is why one of the essential rules of science states *"all observations of physical reality are correct, but only within a certain space-time frame."* Strictly speaking, Nature does not know separateness because nothing exists in an autonomous state. Apparent conflicts in Nature are artificial, merely products of the human mind that arise because individual scientists *have chosen* to study similar aspects of nature in different ways using different methods. Scientists are aware of the potential dangers of this methodological illusion; they recognize the need for continually revising and integrating of all pertinent knowledge so that our view and understanding of Nature will be more complete and more efficiently utilized in our daily lives.

How does this apply to medicine? Conventional medicine *has chosen* to study laws and phenomena of Nature as they are expressed in Man through the study and application of a chemico-pharmaceutical paradigm. Homeopathy, on the other hand, *has chosen* to study the same laws and phenomena, but through the analysis and application of Man's energetic level of being. While conventional medicine reduces and divides Man into separate diseased organs, based upon superficial chemico-structural abnormalities, homeopathy views the pathological involvement of different organs and systems in an ill person as interconnected phases of one whole abnormal energetic state. There is no reason for conflict between the conventional and homeopathic paradigms; any complex system of interconnecting parts contains many levels of functioning. The only way a conflict may arise is if scientists, engineers, or doctors choose to ignore information and fail to revise and integrate the available body of knowledge.

If you were an aircraft engineer, who failed to integrate the numerous components of your craft (based on the corresponding laws, disciplines or phenomena of science, i.e., aerodynamics, electromagnetism, resonance, law of gravity, material engineering, etc.) your plane could malfunction or even crash. In such a case, neglecting "to build staircases" between all pertinent knowledge could be disastrous. American medicine, unlike the numerous branches of the manufacturing sector, where deviations from the rule of information integration would inevitably result in staggering financial or even criminal liabilities, has neglected to apply this principle in the management of the most complex and undoubtedly mysterious "machine" of all—Man. Furthermore, there is no designated body that exists within mainstream medicine to oversee or concern itself with the integration of all available information into medical practice. If anything, just the opposite. In the majority of states, medical licensing boards follow strict laws that threaten to revoke the professional licenses of physicians who deviate from "standard medical practices" (i.e., drugs and surgeries) no matter how successful and scientifically sound alternative approaches might be.

How would one "build a staircase" and integrate homeopathy, based on energy dynamics, with conventional medicine, which is based on body chemistry? According to the rules of science, the more fundamental level of analysis is recognized as the more important. "More fundamental" means that the laws of Nature operating at that level encompass and explain "less fundamental" levels of analysis.

Q: How does physics rank homeopathy and conventional pharmacology?
A: In short, physics states that the electromagnetic interactions between elementary, subatomic particles produce fields and forces that govern chemistry and chemical reactions. These interactions are described by quantum electrodynamics, which has established that without stable quantum energetics there would be no chemistry because matter would disintegrate into subatomic chaos.

Throughout the past century, a number of respected scientists have addressed the failure of conventional medicine and mainstream biology to incorporate a broad spectrum of human energy-based approaches in their research and medical practice. This had been suggested by the world renowned Dutch physicist and Nobel Prize winner, Niels Bohr, 70 years ago.

Professor Murray Gell-Mann has written, "The laws of elementary particle physics are valid, for all matter, throughout the universe, under all conditions. I know of no serious scientist who believes that there are special chemical forces that do not arise from underlying physical forces: Chemistry is the upshot of Elementary Particle Physics."[144]

Austrian physicist Erwin Schrödinger, another Nobel Laureate has agreed: "Chemical reactions are governed by special physical forces of quantum electrodynamics."[145]

Furthermore, Professor M.V. Volkenstein, Director of the Institute of Molecular Biology of the Academy of Science of the former USSR, has attested that: "Every natural science has many levels of investigation and the deepest level is always physical. An exclusion of physics from biology is non-constructive and non-scientific."[146]

In his essay, "Toward a Future Medicine Based on Controlled Energy Fields", Stanford University Professor William A. Tiller observed that conventional medicine addresses illness only at the most superficial level.[147] He sees the first and second levels as energetic, relating to the cause of disease and extent of cellular memory; with the third level, the superficial level, the biochemical abnormalities have resulted from disturbances in the first two levels. In contrast, homeopathy addresses all three levels of illness.

As described in the scientific classic, *Living Systems,* a major scientific flaw of conventional medicine stems from its exclusion of physics and the related fundamental and governing principles from the practice of modern medicine. This was the conclusion of a large group of multidisciplinary scientists from around the world, internationally recognized in their respective specialties. It should be noted that none of these prominent scientists could be identified as an advocate of alternative medicine.[148]

The following examples demonstrate the importance and benefits of addressing diseases on a fundamental level. In each case, a reversal of very serious pathologies was achieved without resorting to invasive and expensive interventions.

- *A teenage girl was scheduled for surgery for a bleeding breast tumor. An acupuncturist chose not to treat her breast per se, but instead focused on a few sore points on the girl's shins that were related to an old injury. Within two weeks the breast tumor disappeared and the surgery became obsolete.*[149]
- *A 35-year old woman had a large ovarian tumor that could be only partially removed. Many abdominal lymph nodes were affected by metastases. From the conventional oncological standpoint, the case was incurable. Nevertheless, chemotherapy and radiation therapy were offered. The patient refused and selected homeopathy instead. She was treated with two principal reme-*

dies: Viburnum prunifolium, *a remedy with high affinity for ovarian tumors and Carcinosin, a homeopathic cancer vaccine prepared from cancerous tissue. Seven years later, repeated CAT scans showed no evidence of tumor and the woman reported feeling healthy.*[150]

◆ *A 37-year-old woman suffered from a recurrent brain tumor in spite of several brain surgeries. She was treated with several homeopathic remedies on a rotating basis and recovered completely. A brain CAT scan confirmed that the tumor had completely disappeared. More than 10-years later there was no evidence of tumor recurrence.*[151]

◆ *A man in his forties suffered from severe congestive heart failure due to a mysterious disease of the heart muscle. His heart contraction was poor, only 15% (normal is 50–70%). In spite of taking as many as 10 pharmaceuticals daily, including a high dose of diuretic that he was placed on at a university hospital, his lifestyle remained poor. He was disabled, pale, weak, and became short of breath after walking only a few blocks. He was also depressed as he could not support his family and was aware that he did not have long to live. Statistics for survival in cases like his are poor.*

Within a short period of homeopathic treatment, his quality of life improved drastically. He regained much energy and was able to quadruple his walking distance without any breathing difficulty at all. He was able to discontinue the diuretic, and decrease the total number of his daily pharmaceuticals from 10 to 4. In addition, a heart test confirmed objectively that heart contractility had more than doubled in strength.

In all likelihood, the patient would have made further progress on the homeopathic therapy if his university hospital cardiologist had not convinced him to discontinue homeopathic treatment because homeopathy, in his opinion, was just a "placebo treatment."

◆ *A college student who was being treated for bad acne was told by her endocrinologist that she would have to live with the condition unless she took hormones daily because a blood test had showed that her body was overproducing testosterone.*

Instead of addressing this problem on a chemical level with hormonal pharmaceuticals and risking their inevitable side ef-fects, she was treated with the homeopathic remedy Sepia, which was indicated in her case. The acne all but disappeared and her testosterone level became normal.

• *A middle-aged woman came to the office in a state of panic. She had developed persistent enlargement of the lymph nodes in her armpits, and lumps in her breasts. Conventional specialists had urged her to consent to an immediate biopsy as the lymph nodes might be cancerous.*

When asked what event preceded the onset of this condition, she replied it was her mother's death from cancer some months prior. Mourning itself was only a part of the problem. The woman had not had the chance to resolve a serious matter with her mother before her death.

She had meant to approach her father on this same very painful issue, but also was unable to do so before his death. She wanted to know if her parents had ever loved her for who she was. She had tried to earn their love throughout her life by obeying their constant demands and suppressing her own emotional needs.

This had tormented her, yet she lacked the courage to confront them when they were still alive.

Assessment: patient pleasant, timid with self-doubt; fears as-serting herself and confronting others. The lymph node enlarge-ment was perhaps the compensatory outlet for her protracted grief and repressed emotions.

These psycho-somatic characteristics are well-matched with the field-state of the remedy Staphysagria. It was administered in high potency, 1M, one pellet.

On follow-up, all of her enlarged lymph nodes and breast lumps had vanished. The emotional relief was no less dramatic. "I feel happy and relieved," she said. "This torture has finally come to an end."

Appendix to Chapter 2

The dichotomy between conventional medicine's seemingly rigorous scientific research and its therapeutic ineffectiveness is puzzling. As a disenchanted allopathic physician once wrote, *"Who among us has not repeatedly seen claims of fourth-generation drugs with no side effects, new operations that yield glowing results with minimal complications, or the latest infallible, high-tech diagnostic procedure, only to discover months or years later that these claims missed the truth by miles?"*[152]

To better understand the roots of this dichotomy, we need to look at the *scientific discovery process* which lies at the heart of any research, including bio-medical research.[153]

This process consists of four main stages:

1. **Induction**
   Scientists conceive of an idea they wish to investigate, based upon some prior observation or hypothesis. This idea may arise within already established scientific disciplines, such as a biochemical process that lead to the manufacture of a new drug, or may spawn a new framework, as in the discovery of the structure of DNA.
2. **Analysis**
   Scientists analyze the facts and tools at their disposal in order to design an experiment that would investigate their idea.
3. **Experiment**
   Scientists test the idea.
4. **Results**
   Scientists examine their observations and determine whether the results they have obtained are positive or negative, statistically significant or not.

From this brief presentation, it becomes very clear that if certain factors or considerations are omitted, either intentionally or from a lack of awareness, on the first two stages of the scientific discovery process, then neither the experiment nor the results will be able to correct omissions.

In other words, the "discovery" in question will automatically inherit all of the assets or liabilities contained within the two initial stages. Both the assets and the shortcomings will become part of the world of medical practice. The more encompassing and inclusive the initial two stages, the more the results will be meaningful and capable of addressing complex and difficult problems.

Of course, it is not a goal of every experiment to determine complex solutions to complex problems. A simple experiment can be of practical significance so long as its findings are integrated into a body of existing knowledge.

The discoveries of science also have their own hierarchical values. There are some, such as the law of gravity and principles of electromagnetism, which are highly revered and which establish their own unique level within the "staircase" of science. Some discoveries, indeed, are of the highest value, such as Einstein's *Theory of Relativity*. The work of an unimaginable human genius, it not only established the existence of another level of Nature, but also transcended and unified several other levels. On the other hand, there have been plenty of discoveries that have added very little in the way of *important* knowledge.

It is easy to see how the prevailing biomedical research models remain oblivious to the inclusion of the energy-related level in their experiments, and produce mainly "amputated" solutions. For example, if drug "A" appears to be a partial solution to problem "A" (i.e., hypertension), it will be recommended as an effective treatment and "latest discovery." Formally, it is correct. However, it may be that problem A can be prevented or completely resolved much more quickly and less expensively by means of body energy-based interventions. But these cannot be "discovered" unless the possibility of their existence is considered during stages one and two of the scientific discovery process.

What is established as the end result of conventionally-oriented research? Unassailable solutions, or "scientifically proven" best ways to remedy hypertension, Parkinson's disease or cancer? No. Only some partial benefits, along with limitations and side effects from the use of drugs for the treatment of hypertension, Parkinson's disease or cancer. Financial pressures often dictate that research will focus on drug development rather than on healing. The same limitations beset the majority of allopathic diagnostic and therapeutic procedures. While all yield some benefit, they fall far short of being the best of available medical options. Worse, experience has shown that a drug's effectiveness declines over time. Consequently, because the drug is not a cure and cannot address true causes of the illness, the patient worsens gradually while the existing causes further erode the body's reserves. Thus, more diseases emerge, more drugs become necessary, and the patient often becomes crippled with side effects.

This is why we can evaluate news of another medical discovery or breakthrough objectively only with the full understanding of the research model that gave birth to the discovery. Otherwise we lose sight of how medical science, driven mainly by proprietary interests, to quote Professor Becker, "becomes our enemy instead of our friend." Through ignorance, we run the risk of being duped by pseudoscientific hoopla and brainwashing.

> *For example, Mrs. D, a patient of mine, was very distraught because her husband had just been diagnosed with prostate cancer. She also was displeased with the office staff of the urologist treating him. She and her husband, however, were reluctant to consult a different urologist or consider other alternatives because this urologist was listed by a very reputable newspaper as one of the "top ten" prostate cancer specialists in the U.S. Unfortunately, this specialist had not been able to decrease Mr. D's very high serum prostate specific antigen (PSA) concentration (a biomarker of the severity of prostate disease) during the previous three years. He was able neither to reverse the process while it was still in its mild form nor prevent its progression toward malignant transformation.*

Yet, only one of the many examples from my practice demonstrates a far better response to the same problem. A man in his mid-fifties who presented with an elevated PSA, double the upper normal value, had it go down three-fold to normal range thanks to the digital medicine approach.

The question is: Did the well-known newspaper grossly mislead its readers? Officially, no; the urologist was indeed reputed to be among the "top ten" in his field. But the ranking could not overcome the limitations of *allopathic paradigm of practice.* Only when this aspect is taken into consideration can the specialist's *overall* expertise be evaluated properly.

Chapter 3

Is Homeopathy Capable of Treating and Preventing Serious Infectious Diseases?

A large body of data demonstrates the potential for homeopathic remedies to be effective and to offer preventatives to populations threatened with biological terrorism. Homeopathic medicine offers the means by which to contain the ravages of deadly infectious epidemics, including smallpox, the most feared agent of our time. Examples follow.

Plague and Scarlet Fever

As a historical fact, and almost 300 years prior to Dr. Hahnemann's production of the first homeopathic remedy, Theophrastus Paracelsus, MD, was reputed to have cured many persons afflicted with a deadly plague by applying the homeopathic principle, *"same cures same."* To prepare his remedies, he did not use serial dilution and succussion as Hahnemann would. He simply applied a minuscule amount of his patients' own infected mucus, barely sufficient to cover the point of a needle, to a few crumbs of bread, which his patients swallowed. This treatment was similar to the modern administration of a live vaccine.

During the scarlet fever epidemic in Europe in the summer of 1801, Hahnemann observed that in the only two members of a large family who were spared were children taking the *Belladonna* remedy he had prescribed for an unrelated problem some weeks earlier. He was surprised, but when he compared the effects of homeopathic *Belladonna* on a healthy person with the symptoms of scarlet fever, he found homeopathic *Belladonna* produced very high fever, an excruciatingly painful and swollen throat with an intense burning sensation and inability to swallow, deep chills, smooth red skin rash

and enlarged glands. He perceived that *Belladonna* was a homeopathic *Epidemic similimum* or *genus epidemicus* of scarlet fever and
recommended that medical professionals administer it as both prophylaxis and as acute treatment against the disease. Decades later,
official medical statistics confirmed the prudence of his advice.
Homeopathic *Belladonna* had proven to be very successful in the
treatment and prevention of scarlet fever.[154,155]

Typhus

In 1813, following the defeat of Napoleon's army after a three-
day battle in Leipzig, a terrible epidemic of typhoid broke out
among the French soldiers. Hahnemann personally treated 180 of
these cases with homeopathy and, impressively, lost only one patient.[156]

Cholera

In 1831, a deadly epidemic of cholera was spreading rapidly
across Western Europe. Hahnemann noticed two dominant sets of
symptoms in infected individuals: burning fever and severe chills,
alternating with severe diarrhea and constipation. Hahnemann determined that camphor, administered as an *epidemicus similimum,*
produced a similar effect on a healthy person. He suggested that
crude camphor, wherever it was available, be administered in a very
diluted form as both prevention and treatment. With this homeopathic treatment, the mortality rate with this homeopathic treatment
ranged between 2.4% and 21%, while it was over 50% for those
treated conventionally.[157]

Similarly, during the United States' cholera epidemic of 1849,
homeopathic physicians reported that of more than 1,110 people
treated with *Camphor* and other homeopathic remedies in Cincin-
nati, Ohio, they lost only 3%. The mortality rates under conventional, allopathic care were between 40% and 70%.[158] To increase
the credibility of their reports, homeopathic doctors published the
names and addresses of all of the patients who had survived or died
in a local newspaper. The American Medical Association de-
nounced the findings from what it termed, a "society of quackery,"
but local conventional physicians declared that homeopathic
Camphor was one of the most valuable remedies for patients

with cholera and then extended full credit to their homeopathic colleagues.[159]

Yellow Fever

Homeopathy is also credited with successful treatment of the serious yellow fever epidemic that raged through the southern United States in 1878. Again, mortality figures among patients treated by homeopathy were about one-third that of the patients who were treated conventionally. Even conventional medical experts acknowledged the value of homeopathic remedies in stemming the epidemic.[160]

Smallpox

In 1902, during a deadly smallpox epidemic in Iowa, homeopathy came to the rescue again. More than 2,800 persons, 547 of whom were known to have already been exposed to smallpox, were immunized by 15 homeopathic doctors with the homeopathic remedy *Variolinum*, prepared from an infected smallpox skin blister. Of the patients who received the remedy, only 13 developed smallpox symptoms.[161] This homeopathic treatment was supported and upheld by a ruling by the Iowa State Supreme Court.

In another instance, a homeopathic physician vaccinated two hundred school children with *Variolinum,* and a large number of them developed vaccine response symptoms similar to those that generally follow the administration of the conventional smallpox vaccine. This suggested that the homeopathic remedy had indeed induced immune responses energetically, despite the absence of a physical virus.[162]

Polio

Arthur Hill Grimmer, MD, a prominent homeopathic physician, conducted a clinical trial in his private practice in the early 1950's. During the polio epidemic in the U.S., Grimmer tested the *genus epidemicus* remedy, *Lathyrus sativa,* made from chickpeas, as a preventative. Chickpeas had been known to cause severe and persistent paralysis of the legs if consumed frequently in large amounts. For example, during a wheat famine in India, when the flour of chickpeas was used instead of wheat flour to make bread, many people developed permanent paralysis of the lower limbs. Polio is also known to induce various degrees of paralysis of the lower extremities. Grimmer administered *Lathyrus sativa* to both children and adults in gradually increasing potency a few times a year for up to five years. He reported a 100% success rate in preventing polio.[163]

In 1957, Dr. Grimmer's method was put to the test by Argentinian homeopaths during a polio epidemic in Buenos Aires. Thousands of people were placed on his protocol for homeopathic prevention. A 100% success rate again was reported.[164] Between 1956 and 1961, *Lathyrus sativa* in high potencies was administered to more than 50,000 people worldwide. Only one subject developed symptoms of polio. In that case the symptoms developed one day after ingesting a dose of *Lathyrus sativa* and were non-paralytic.[165]

Meningitis

In 1974, during a meningococcal meningitis epidemic in Brazil, 18,640 children were vaccinated with one-low-potency dose of *Meningococcinum,* a homeopathic remedy prepared from meningococcus bacteria taken in one low potency dose. Only four children developed meningitis, compared to 32 reported cases among 6,340 "control" children who did not receive the remedy.[166]

Whooping Cough

In a study of the homeopathic whooping cough remedy, *Pertussinum,* prepared from infected mucus containing pertussis bacteria, significantly reduced the severity of the disease.[167]

Tularemia

In 1991 for a study of serious Tularemia infection, a group of mice was given a homeopathic isode prepared from *Francisella tularensis,* the infectious agent causing the disease. After all the mice had been infected with the actual agent, a statistically significant decreased rate of infection was achieved, compared to placebo-treated mice.[168]

Diphtheria

In France in 1932, the homeopathic isode, *Diphtherinum,* prepared from an infectious agent causing diphtheria, was given as an immunization to 45 children. Every child developed circulating antibodies against diphtheria (confirming that this remedy had appropriately stimulated immune responses). Several years later, as the children's antibody levels declined, *Diphtherinum* was readministered and restored the high antibody concentrations.[169] In two other studies, prophylaxis of diphtheria with *Diphtherinum* produced positive immunization in over 60% of immunized children.[170,171]

Malaria

In 1993, doctors at the University of Amsterdam conducted two studies of homeopathic treatment of malaria during an epidemic in Ghana, Africa. Homeopathic treatment proved to be as effective as chloroquine, a conventional drug for malaria. Unfortunately, the small size of the study group precluded definitively demonstrating the superiority of the homeopathic remedy over chloroquine.[172]

As an Alternative to Childhood Vaccinations

Isaac Golden, PhD, ND, recently concluded a 10-year clinical study in Australia of the efficacy of homeopathic preventative remedies for childhood diphtheria, haemophilus bacteria, measles, mumps, polio, tetanus and whooping cough. The remedies were administered on a rotating basis, beginning at one month of age, and continuing for the first five years of life. Out of 1,305 participating families, about 70% of the parents returned detailed questionnaires concerning their children's responses, side effects, and overall health. On average, only 11% of the children contracted any of these infections, compared to typical infection rates of 5% to 25% among similar children immunized with conventional vaccines. Mild and transient side effects occurred in only 10% of the children immunized homeopathically (long-term complications are known to occur with conventional vaccines). The overall health of these homeopathically-vaccinated children was considered to be excellent and much better than the health of their allopathically-vaccinated peers.[173]

AIDS

In 1990, Belgian doctors published the results of a placebo-controlled study conducted in Zaire, Africa, concerning the treatment of patients with symptomatic acquired immunodeficiency syndrome

(AIDS). One group of patients was given a complex homeopathic preparation that consisted of several remedies. After two years, the homeopathically treated group registered significantly less weight loss, decreased frequency of fever and diarrhea, and enjoyed a lower mortality rate.[174]

In 1996, the results of a double-blind placebo-controlled study performed at the Bastyr University Naturopathic College of Medicine in Seattle, Washington, demonstrated positive effects of homeopathic remedies in very high potencies for AIDS patients The remedies were prepared from several physiological hormonal growth factors known to stimulate various immune system and blood elements. Compared to the effects of the placebo, the remedies produced a statistically greater improvement of the immune system and blood elements, increased weight gain, and decreased viral load.[175]

Lyme Disease

There was an interesting report published in the official Journal of the National Center of Homeopathy, *Homeopathy Today,* by a veterinary physician from Connecticut regarding homeopathic treatment and prevention of Lyme disease. Over a five-year period, he has placed more than five hundred cats, dogs and horses on a homeopathic immunization program with a remedy prepared from *Borrellia burgdorferi,* the spirochete that causes Lyme disease. Only two dogs appeared to have contracted Lyme disease following the homeopathic immunization, and these two were promptly cured with a homeopathic remedy. In contrast, according to a Cornell Veterinary School Diagnostic Lab study, almost one-third (32%) of dogs vaccinated with conventional vaccine, contracted Lyme disease despite vaccination and over half became infected as the direct result of the vaccine.[176]

Overall Effectiveness in Human Epidemics

In a review published in 1900, the overall death rates per 100 patients in homeopathic hospitals in the U.S. during epidemics were from one-half to one-eighth as low as those reported in conventional medical hospitals.[177]

Chapter 4

Is Homeopathy Capable of Protecting Against and Treating the Consequences of Toxicological Agents and Chemical Warfare?

Numerous research studies have been performed on experimental animals, cell cultures and plants in order to explore the effectiveness of homeopathic remedies in cases of poisoning. In most of these experiments, the remedies tested have been homeopathic preparations of the offending agents, isodes.

These experiments and the experience of thousands of homeopathic practitioners worldwide who successfully use toxicological isodes to treat their patients, have demonstrated their immense effectiveness. Their potential in the treatment of acute and chronic ailments following chemical warfare cannot be overestimated. The author also shares his own experience throughout this book via clinical examples of the use of these indispensable therapeutic agents in routine medical care.

In our turbulent times, there is a dire therapeutic need for utilization of toxicological isodes in cases of medical emergencies born out of chemical warfare, accidents, and general pollution and even under the circumstances of hostage rescue operations where noxious pharmacological airborne agents have to be used. The most recent example is the Russian rescue operation of October 2002 in a Moscow theater where over a hundred hostages died as the result of the use of fentanyl, a strong narcoleptic gas. Without a doubt that the casualties would have been minimal had the hostages been afforded the homeopathic fentanyl promptly.

The following studies illustrate the successful use of homeopathic remedies against toxicological agents:

Arsenic

In separate experiments using rats, guinea pigs and pigeons, successful detoxification of arsenic with homeopathic arsenic preparations was demonstrated.[178]

Bismuth

The researchers who studied arsenic also demonstrated successful detoxification of another toxic metal, bismuth, in rats given homeopathic isodes of bismuth. In order to test the specificity of homeopathic isodes, arsenic poisoned rats were treated with homeopathic bismuth and rats poisoned with bismuth received homeopathic arsenic. There was no therapeutic effect or increase in urinary secretions of either metal under these circumstances, confirming the need for therapeutic specificity in the use of homeopathic remedies.[179–181]

Cadmium

Homeopathic cadmium proved effective in reducing mortality in frogs intoxicated with cadmium.[182] In a separate study, homeopathic cadmium protected kidney cell cultures from cadmium-induced damage.[183]

Lead

Homeopathic lead was found to prevent liver damage in rats poisoned with lead.[184] However, this effect was not reproducible.[185] In the experience of this author, a choice of a proper potency will often determine the effectiveness of homeopathic isodes.

Copper

Plants previously exposed to toxic doses of copper salt recovered completely when given homeopathic copper salt.[186]

Mercury

In six independent placebo-controlled studies of mercury intoxicated rodents, homeopathic mercury significantly reduced mortality.[187–189]

Pesticides

Fifty cases of cats and dogs accidentally poisoned by either arsenic metal or the toxic compounds, metaldehyde or organophosphorus, contained in pesticides, have been reported from a homeopathic veterinary practice. All pets fell ill with signs of significant neurotoxicity, including repetitive seizures. In serious cases, the average mortality under conventional veterinary treatment is 50% and prolonged treatment with hospitalizations is the rule. Of the 50 pets treated with the homeopathic remedy, *Arsenicum album,* prepared from arsenic, only 4 deaths occurred—a mortality rate of only 8%. In addition, 80% of the remaining 46 pets returned home within 12 hours after initiation of homeopathic treatment; within 24 hours, all of the 46 surviving pets had gone home. None of the 46 survivors sustained any residual health impairment.[190]

Tetrachloride

Rats poisoned with tetrachloride, a highly toxic agent causing degeneration of normal liver cells into fibrotic or scar tissue, developed hepatic inflammation, fibrosis and elevated serum liver enzyme activities, reflecting liver damage. They were then given a 30C potency dilution of the homeopathic remedy, *Phosphorus,* which is known for its effect in protecting the liver in humans. Homeopathic treatment produced a reduction of elevated liver enzymes and complete protection from hepatic fibrosis.[191–197]

Alloxan

Alloxan is known to cause diabetes by killing the insulin-producing cells of the pancreas. When homeopathic *Alloxan 9C* was given to mice before and after alloxan administration, pancreatic damage either did not occur at all, or in the unprotected group where it had already taken place, it was reversed after *Alloxan 9C* was administered.[198]

Carcinogens

The carcinogenic substances 2-acetylaminofluorene and phenobarbital, known to cause liver cancer, were ingested by rats as part of their daily diet. The addition of homeopathic isodes to these carcinogens in their drinking water significantly reduced the incidence of chemically-induced liver cancer and delayed the progression of those tumors that had already occurred. In contrast, a nonspecific homeopathic remedy was not protective.[199]

The carcinogenic chemotherapy drugs, nalixidine and cisplatin, were given to live cell cultures that had been pre-treated with the corresponding homeopathic isodes. A significantly reduced incidence of drug-induced carcinogenesis was observed.[200,201]

Poisonous Mushroom

Lethal doses of a poison produced by the toxic mushroom, *Amanita phaloides,* were administered to rats followed by the homeopathic isode of the same poison. The homeopathic remedy significantly reduced the toxicity of the poison.[202]

Poisonous Plants

Two poisonous plants, *Aconite* and *Veratrum,* each containing toxic alkaloids, induced life-threatening heart fibrillation in animal experiments. Pretreatment with either homeopathic *Aconite* or homeopathic *Veratrum,* as appropriate, were significantly cardioprotective.[203]

Chemical Warfare

In anticipation of a German mustard gas attack during World War II, the British government studied the potentially protective effect of homeopathic mustard gas. This remedy exhibited positive prophylactic and therapeutic effects.[204]

Ionizing Radiation

Mice treated with protective homeopathic remedies *(Ginseng; Ruta graveolens)* before and after being subjected to high doses of radiation exhibited significantly greater protection from radiation damage than did mice treated with an irrelevant homeopathic remedy.[205,206]

Snake venom

A lethal snake venom was given to mice, who proved to be protected by the homeopathic isode of the same snake venom.[207]

Toxic Drug

Gentamycin, an antibiotic known for its highly toxic effects on the kidneys, was injected into rats. Homeopathic gentamycin isode was reno-protective.[208]

Summary of Homeopathic Toxicology and postulated mechanisms of protective action

There were 135 studies published between 1955 and 1993 that investigated the potential protective effects of homeopathic remedies. Most of the remedies studied were isodes. Review and evaluation of these studies by an independent team of researchers from the Walter Reed Army Institute of Research in Washington, D.C., and three university centers in Germany, concluded that in more than 70% of these studies, the research was of good quality and positive outcomes were supported by rigorous statistical analysis. Interestingly, the strongest evidence was demonstrated by those studies where the highest dilutions were used, that is, when the remedy had been diluted far beyond the presence of even a single molecule remaining of the original substance. By purely conventional pharmacological criteria, these preparations had to be completely inert and devoid of any biological activity or action, yet they produced statistically significant outcomes. The reviewers concluded that there was sufficient evidence to justify the consideration of homeopathic preparations for protection in cases of toxic exposure.

It was postulated that homeopathic remedies may confer disease resistance by inducing a chronic immune stress response. This effect closely resembles that of conventional vaccines, where the immune stress response is known to elicit long-lasting effects.[209]

Another hypothesis concerns the already mentioned gating theory, whereby cells become "deaf" to the actions of offending agents.

Other Beneficial Effects

Metabolic Problems

A state of **thyrotoxicosis**—hyperactive thyroid crisis, a potentially life endangering condition—was induced in experimental animals. Treatment with homeopathic thyroid hormone was curative.[210]

Histamine, known to produce severe swelling and inflammation, was injected into rats. (Many pharmaceutical drugs aimed at containment of allergic reactions contain histamine blockers.) Homeopathic histamine aborted inflammation.[211]

Aspirin is known to prolong bleeding time and to cause potentially fatal hemorrhaging in humans. In contrast, homeopathic aspirin shortened bleeding time in healthy human volunteers.[212]

High serum total cholesterol concentration in rabbits was significantly reduced by the homeopathic remedy, *Chelidonium,* in *3X* potency. *Chelidonium* is known to affect the liver, gall bladder and bile, all known to be involved in cholesterol metabolism.[213]

The homeopathic remedies, *Gelsemium sempervirens, Cannabis indica, Graphites* and *Agaricus muscaris,* induce nerve blockade resulting in motor paralysis in healthy animals. In neurological diseases, they are as effective as the conventional drugs, *pilocarpine* and *aloperidol,* in the reversal of neurological blocks.[214–217]

Protection Against Heat Shock

Pretreatment with a homeopathic remedy to protect against heat shock significantly increased the resistance of live cell cultures.[218]

Positive Effects on the Immune System

Immuno-compromised mice demonstrated significant stimulation of cellular and humoral immune functions, in response to a homeopathic preparation of the thymus gland and its hormone, *thymulin.*[219–224]

Circulating concentrations of the antiviral and antitumorogenic glycoproteins, the *interferons,* increased in response to homeopathic α- and β-interferons.[225]

The homeopathic remedy, *Silicea,* widely used to expedite recovery in chronic infections and poorly healing wounds, significantly increased the immune response and accelerated the healing of open wounds in rodents.[226,227]

Immune response was restored to immunodeficient chick embryos by treatment with homeopathic *bursin,* the avian equivalent of the human thymus hormone, *thymulin.* Pituitary and adrenal function also increased.[228–230]

A multi-national study conducted at universities in Canada, France, Israel and Italy demonstrated enhanced cell-mediated immunity in humans who received a homeopathic remedy prepared from antibodies to human immunoglobulin.[231]

Chapter 5

Environmental Pollution in the Aftermath of September 11 and the Diagnostic and Therapeutic Limitations of Conventional Medicine

The burning and collapse of the gigantic towers of the World Trade Center released large amounts of some of the world's most toxic substances into the environment, including *asbestos, benzene, dioxin, fiberglass, mercury, lead, PCB's, silicon and sulfuric acid.* Most of these agents are known to cause cancer, severe lung pathology, neurological and cardiovascular disease and a myriad of immune dysfunctions. Among the people exposed were many whose health was compromised already from living in a highly polluted environment. Undoubtedly, the environmental impact of the towers' collapse increased many people's risk for developing serious health ailments. This is especially of concern for pregnant and nursing mothers, and their children.

Yet, this troubling situation should be taken with context: The majority of "healthy" people in the industrialized nations, particularly in the big cities, are mobile containers of toxic pollutants with as many as 100 pollutants documented to reside within human tissues.[232] According to the Environmental Protection Agency (EPA), traces of toxic chemicals can be found in nearly every American.[233] Many of these agents are known carcinogens. According to the National Cancer Institute (NCI), up to 98% of all cancers may be linked to chemical exposures.[234–240]

While the "clean-air subcommittee" chaired by U.S. senators Hilary Clinton (D-NY) and Joseph Lieberman (D-CT) focused in February 2002 on the EPA's examination of the state of air pollution of New York City's outdoor and indoor environments after September 11, the more pertinent question might be: What is the status of these pollutants inside the organs of individual children and adults? The EPA was criticized for producing "wishful data" because the only real medical issue—the presence and levels of these pollutants within human bodies—was not addressed. And although the sub-committee issued a seemingly reassuring and correct recommendation "of a need for long-term health monitoring," whether or not physicians will assume responsibility for this task remains a big question.

The real facts suggest that conventional medicine is incapable of handling toxicological problems for several major reasons:

- On average, physicians in the U.S. receive only a few hours at most of training in toxicology or environmental medicine.[241,242]
- Most of the data concerning public "safe levels" in the environment are based on very limited animal models. These models are inadequate to extrapolate conclusive and accurate standards for humans, who are known for their significant diversity in genetic makeup, state of health, nutritional status, age, pre-existing medical ailments, and medication regimens. All of these factors are known to affect individual resistance to environmental pollutants and their metabolism, which can fluctuate day by day, even in the same person.
- The effects of combined exposure to the 70,000 different chemical compounds that are in common use today in the U.S. are impossible to study or ascertain.[243–248]
- Most chemical toxins do not reside in the blood or other easily accessible body parts, after acute immediate exposure. They are scattered throughout the internal organs, which are practically impossible to access for medical screening purposes. Even when a chemical is found in the blood or other tissue specimens, its concentration often falls into "within normal range" values. There are two major misconceptions operating here. One is that a "convenient specimen" is a "useful specimen." It is important to stress that the composition of an easily accessible specimen may not reflect the true danger to one's health because toxins usually reside more deeply within the body and often prove to be different from the ones obtained in the "convenient specimen."[249] The other is that so called "normal levels" are normal. They are, in fact, fallacies devised by health department bureaucrats who assume that an average urban resident is expected to be "loaded" with a cer-

tain amount of pollutants.[250] Unfortunately, "normal" often translates automatically into "safe" in the minds of physicians and the general public. In addition, conventional medicine is generally unable to recognize and diagnose toxicological problems and their insidious impact on health. Consequently, the carriers of "safe" amounts of environmental toxins are neither "normal" nor "healthy."[251,252] As a result, the only reliable method of establishing a proper determination of the toxin load of an individual, according to the conclusion reached by 120 world-leading toxicologists, is a . . . "post-mortem examination."[253]

* Conventional medicine practically lacks the means of effectively treating chronic chemical intoxications. A few well-known examples to this are the Gulf War Syndrome and "Ground Zero" victims.

* Here again, the use of homeopathic toxicological isodes guided by the diagnostic test presented in the next chapter, becomes indispensable.

Chapter 6

Do Better Diagnostic Tests Exist in Alternative Medicine to Detect Toxicological, Biological and Nuclear Agents?

Do better diagnostic tests exist to detect toxicological, biological and nuclear agents? Fortunately, yes. An alternative diagnostic approach is available that is noninvasive, painless, harmless and simple. This approach is based upon the physiological energetic properties of the human body. Because of these properties, humans possess an uncanny ability to perceive and react to the unique energy field and natural resonant frequency of any substance to which they may be subjected during diagnostic testing.

The underlying mechanisms behind this diagnostic approach are similar to those that have been in wide use in conventional medicine's high-technology procedures, such as electrocardiography (ECG), electroencephalography (EEG), electromyography (EMG), magnetic resonance imaging (MRI), and others. All of these are based on the energetic properties of human cells and the neural and electrical interconnectedness that links the skin, muscles, and internal organs.

The relationship between the skin and internal organs is well-known in medicine as *Head's Zones,* named after English neurologist Sir Henry Head, MD, (1861–1940). Dr. Head observed and mapped a very accurate correlation between unhealthy internal organs and certain corresponding areas of the skin that became hypersensitive as the result of their links to these organs. *Head's Zones* are analogous to the relationships between ill organs and their corresponding skin points along the acupuncture meridians that have been known for as long as five thousand years in Chinese medicine.

The first attempt to implement noninvasive testing based upon the reaction of the human body to an energetic field of a substance was made by Albert Abrams, MD, who was the Dean of Clinical

Medicine at Stanford Medical School in the early 1900's. In his experiments, he noticed changes in some physical examination findings that occurred only while patients were touched with a wire that was connected on the other end with either samples of diseased tissue, blood from sick people or bacterial cultures. He believed that a wire was delivering energy of the samples via radio-like waves and named his method as *radionics*. In time, he constructed a simple testing device that was able to test people non-invasively by measuring their physical responses after subjecting them to the numerous pathological samples or biological agents.

His method became popular in Europe and was even reviewed by the Royal Society of Medicine of Great Britain in 1922. Despite 25 successful trials, with the odds of this happening by chance being 1 in 33,554,432, the society acceded this and suggested "a very high degree of probability" but declined to sanction this method or introduce it into medical mainstream.[254] In the U.S., Head and his method have been dismissed as quackery by the medical establishment ever since. Yet Sir James Barr, MD, a past president of the British Medical Association, was among many knowledgeable professionals and scientists who successfully reproduced Abram's experiments. Dr. Barr referred to Abrams as one of the greatest medical geniuses who ever lived.[255]

In the 1920's, a group of medical homeopathic doctors confirmed Dr. Abrams' hypothesis that the human body is able to react to the field emitted by a substance. This occurs when the substance is brought into close contact with the skin or placed directly into the patient's hand. Indeed, the body was shown to be capable of distinguishing a harmful substance from a useful substance. This was evidenced by patients' reflex reactions in response to a well-indicated versus an "unwanted" homeopathic remedy. The "correct" remedies elicited several positive involuntary responses of the autonomic nervous system caused by changes in the electrical conductance of the skin. Among these were skin circulation, pupil reaction, color change in the iris of the eye and decrease in heart rate. The "wrong" remedies produced different and adverse effects on these physiologic functions.[256]

In the early 1930's, Professor H. Burr and his research group from Yale University built a special apparatus that enabled them to gauge the correlation of voltage between healthy or diseased organs and skin voltage measured over the corresponding areas on the body. Abnormal voltage proved to be highly indicative of underlying organ pathology. A clinical trial conducted in the late 1940's at Bellevue Hospital in New York City verified the accuracy of this approach. The technique correctly diagnosed women known to have uterine cancer. These results were published in the *American Journal of Obstetrics and Gynecology* in 1949.[257–262]

George Crile, Sr., MD, the famous surgeon and researcher in human energy field, became disenchanted with the inability or severe limitations of conventional diagnostic methods and even post-mortem examinations to establish the true causes of chronic diseases. He commented in frustration, that even autopsies "do little more than to say that the patient is dead."

Noting that every pathological process, whether injuries, intoxications, pollutants or infections, always produces corresponding electrical changes in living tissues, he called on the medical community to "test in the clinic the science of radio-electric pathology."[263]

Inspired by the progress achieved in his own research, Crile proclaimed in 1933 that energetic diagnosis had an unlimited potential to detect the most dreadful diseases, perhaps even years before illness appears. He concluded that this field constituted the future of medicine.[264]

"His own received him not", however, and after the deaths of Dr. Crile and Professor Burr, their research in radio-electric diagnosis gathered dust.

Energy-based human diagnosis is based on the electrical properties of our cells. There are at least three different types of innate electrical systems that human cells possess: alternating electric (AC) current, direct continuous (DC) current, and the electromagnetic fields (EMF's) emitted by the atoms of the cells. The presence of the magnetic cellular phenomenon was mentioned earlier. Conventional medicine takes only partial advantage of some of these properties. For example, well-known medical tests, including the electroencephalogram (EEG), electrocardiogram (EKG), and electromyogram (EMG), record AC current in the brain, heart and peripheral muscles, respectively.

The DC current originates from perineural tissue, the sheaths that enclose and protect the cells of the brain and spinal cord as well as the peripheral nerves. The brain, spinal cord, nerves, and surrounding sheaths constitute a major part of a long-range communication system in our bodies.[265,266]

The cellular electromagnetic field system plays a key role in the regulation of physiological processes. The radiations of this system extend beyond our bodies and represent our first line of defense against microbes. For example, certain acupuncture methods that are known to increase the strength of the external or skin energy field, "Qi" ("Chi"), have been demonstrated to increase resistance to infections and disease, even in AIDS patients. This external human energy field has been recorded and photographed by scientists in the former USSR and in the U.S. In the 1980's, Professor Valerie Hunt at UCLA, continuing the work of Professor Burr and Dr. Crile, used sophisticated computerized technology to record the external energy field of humans, plants, and other living organisms. She demonstrated the sensitivity of this field to internal pathology and its changes years before it would be recognized by conventional diagnostic tests.[267] In 1939, Semyon Davidovich Kirlian, Soviet engineer of X-ray technology, built a high frequency photography apparatus that was able to photograph the energy fields of humans, animals and plants and to establish the field patterns of healthy, diseased and cancerous tissues.

Gleb Frank, an academician and Director of Science of the Institute of Biological Physics of the Academy of Science, endorsed the use of Kirlian photography in medical science. Professor S.M. Pavlenko, MD, chairman of the Pathophysiology Department at Moscow Medical Institute, predicted great potential in the use of external energy fields in the early diagnosis of cancer.

In the early 1950's, Reinhold Voll, MD of Germany, was diagnosed with cancer of the urinary bladder and was given by his allopathic colleagues only a few years to live. He went outside of his conventional medical training and the oncological paradigm and undertook a serious study of the energy-related medical specialties, acupuncture and homeopathy. He became fascinated with the fact that each of the 20 acupuncture meridians was known to pass through internal organs and tissues and energetically connects just about all of the human anatomy.

One of the major and longest meridians in the body is known as the *urinary bladder meridian,* whose path originates from the urinary bladder itself. After becoming acquainted with Roger de la Fuye the French doctor, and his book, *"Traite d'Acupuncture" (Treatise on Acupuncture)* concerning therapeutic applications of minimal electric current along meridians for therapeutic organ support, Dr. Voll conceived of the idea of "tuning into" organs through certain acupuncture points along their corresponding acupuncture meridians for diagnostic purposes. Using his knowledge in radio- and electro-engineering, he built an apparatus capable of obtaining skin resistance measurements off the acupuncture points.[268] He first registered normal ranges for the skin resistance of acupuncture points, noting that they were different from the values of skin resistance recorded from the surrounding skin. He then compared them to skin resistance measurements of patients who were known to have pathological involvement of various organs, himself included.

After he established a clear distinction between the readings from healthy and ill persons, he demonstrated his novel method to his medical colleagues, using his own healthy and sick skin points. However, the demonstration started out as a complete embarrassment because his sick points all suddenly measured as normal. He apologized profusely to the audience while searching through his pockets in desperation, hoping that perhaps some electric gadget left in his clothing was throwing off the readings. This was not the case. Instead he came across several homeopathic remedies in his pockets that he had administered to himself. As soon as they were removed, his sick skin points again became abnormal. From this experience, he decided that this communication system may operate in both directions, where organs can sense and confirm effective therapies via skin contact. This may occur through the natural resonant frequencies of medicinal substances, even before they are consumed. Furthermore, some of these substances might be capable of removing the true culprits of acute and chronic diseases. In an attempt to determine the nature of these factors, he created hundreds of miniature testing vials that contained all sorts of environmental pollutants, radioactive materials and biological agents in homeopathic form. Guided by his measurements, he was able to identify the real causes of each organ pathology. He then tested homeopathic isodes and organ support remedies in different potencies in order to determine the most effective therapeutic combination. His applications resulted in many spectacular cures, including that of his own bladder cancer.[269]

Dr. Voll's method, (Electroacupuncture According to Voll; EAV) became very popular, not only in West Germany, but also in Western Europe and Japan. It is estimated that currently there are over 100,000 EAV practitioners worldwide. In Japan, about 40,000 similar devices are in medical use.[270] Dr. Voll was well-recognized in Europe with numerous awards, including a special award from the World Health Organization and a Medal of Honor from the Pope for his monumental contribution to medicine. His discovery opened a new era in Medicine by establishing the true causes of human illnesses non-invasively, painlessly, safely, and inexpensively.

Although EAV inaugurated a new era of *Bio-resonance* diagnosis in medicine, the technique is not fault-free. One drawback is that it requires an extremely laborious and time-consuming process of obtaining hundreds of skin point measurements and then numerous re-measurements for both diagnostic and therapeutic purposes. This makes the test very cumbersome and impractical to utilize in daily practice, particularly in an emergency setting. Some simplified versions of the EAV, such as Vega testing and computerized EAV devices, have failed to solve this and other problems due to the overload of information that these devices are capable of obtaining. There is also the challenge of establishing a clinical hierarchy within this information that would facilitate its effective use in clinical practice.

In 1971, a group of physical therapists in the U.S. presented a textbook of muscle testing and function.[271] Based upon this work and the relationship between individual muscles and acupuncture meridians, George Goodheart, D.C., of Detroit, was able to develop a fairly simple diagnostic technique—*Applied Kinesiology testing (AK)*—which correlates muscle tonus, weak or strong, with the health of the organs with which these muscles communicate via neural pathways.[272,273] Over the years, tens of thousands of health practitioners in the U.S. and abroad have introduced *Applied Kinesiology testing* into their practices.

Skillful practitioners, equipped with homeopathic testing vials identical to the ones used by Dr. Voll, are capable of eliciting valuable medical information by having patients simply hold a vial and then apply pressure to certain muscle groups, checking them for a change in tone. If a muscle exhibits weak tone while the patient is holding a certain vial, then the actual culprit is that agent contained in the vial. With the passage of time, the test has been perfected and simplified. At present, a substance can be placed on a conducting metal platform connected via a conducting cable to a cigar-shaped metal bar and placed into a person's hand during testing. This creates a conductive circuit consisting of the hand, metal bar, connecting cable and platform.

Another important improvement made was that the application of pressure to muscles, in order to elicit a response, was replaced by a simple involuntary muscle reflex displayed by a right lower extremity—positive reading. An absent response would constitute a negative reading. The person would display his response to the testing vials while lying on his back on an examining table or while sitting in a reclining chair.

A practitioner no longer has to test numerous individual muscles in order to identify a weak muscle-organ connection. Instead, a homeopathic organ vial is placed on the platform. If a patient has an underlying problem with that organ, he will react instantly by displaying a positive reading. The culprit behind the weakness or illness of a given organ or tissue can be ascertained further by matching the weak organ or tissue vial against potential offending agents and judged by a positive or negative reading.

A choice of effective therapeutic items also can be promptly determined with Applied Kinesiology testing. In addition, they can be tested for their safety and absence of prohibitive side effects before their administration.

The author has worked to integrate valuable knowledge from both conventional and alternative medical training into this system of Bio-resonance testing, with a particular emphasis on toxicological and biological agents which undoubtedly constitute the true causes of just about all chronic and acute diseases. While conventional medicine merely attempts to contain diseases by identifying pathological findings detected through a myriad of blood and body

chemistry tests, tissue biopsies or imaging tests and then match
these findings with the available pharmaceuticals, without determination of the true causes of disease, skillful practitioners of energy
medicine assume a far better approach. As a rule, these practitioners bypass many of the expensive and not infrequently hazardous
conventional tests and instead identify and remove the cause of disease. This alone often results in its collapse or regression. Because
the body reacts instantly to any testing item whose energy field it
senses, any vial can elicit a response, even those prepared from in-
tra-cellular structures, including DNA. Its rapidity confers unparalleled efficiency to this system of testing; only a few minutes or even
seconds are sufficient to pinpoint the cause of acute or chronic intoxications, infections, emotional or physical traumas or other assaults. The test very much resembles an e-mail communication between the test vials and person's body cells. Even more importantly,
the capability of Bio-resonance testing is unsurpassed in its accuracy and depth of penetration. Actual clinical results vary between
practitioners, who utilize a wide variety of applications of this medical approach and whose success depends on their level of training,
awareness and their choices of therapeutic options.

Bio-resonance testing and the efficacy of the homeopathic therapeutic system have proven to be precise and reliable, as these case
histories attest:

Clinical Cases

A case of plant poisoning

While gardening, a middle-aged man developed severe dermatitis after coming into contact with some poisonous plant. His skin
was covered in many places with huge, nasty red blotches that
itched and burned severely, and his lymph nodes became enlarged.
Because he was exposed to a number of plants, he did not know exactly which was the culprit. He denied the existence of any prior allergies or exposure to poison ivy or poison oak and he did not wish
to go to an emergency room before trying homeopathic treatment
first. I advised him to return to my office along with a sample of
each plant from his garden. He returned with six different plants,
each packed in a separate plastic bag.

Bio-resonance testing identified one of these plants as the culprit. According to the testing, the patient was prescribed the homeopathic isode of the plant in 12K potency, one drop to be taken for two days followed by one dose of the same isode in 200K potency.

Follow-up: Rapid improvement ensued as soon as the treatment began. The patient's symptoms were cured completely within several days.

A case of reversed diabetes

A middle-aged man with Type II Diabetes was receiving a total of 50 units of insulin daily, as prescribed by his diabetes specialist.

Bio-resonance testing discovered the presence of dental metals (silver amalgam and mercury) in many organs, including the pancreas. Homeopathic isodes of silver amalgam and mercury were administered in the potencies determined by testing to be the most therapeutically effective and tolerated, along with proper homeopathic organ support in order to enhance excretion of these metals from the body.

Follow-up: Two weeks following this treatment, the diabetologist discontinued the insulin prescription because the patient's blood sugar concentration was decreasing rapidly. The specialist, however, prescribed an oral diabetes medication because "diabetic patient cannot lose his diabetes."

Bio-resonance testing indicated that oral diabetes drugs would surely cause adverse side effects because pancreatic gland produced a good energetic reading, indicating that the pancreas had returned to healthy function. The drug was discontinued in order to avoid hypoglycemic side effects.

Follow-up: One year later. The blood sugar concentration remained normal and diabetes medications were not required.

A case of reversed diabetes, coronary artery disease and prostate disease

A man in his sixties with recent-onset severe diabetes had experienced a 30-pound weight loss and ketoacidosis which required urgent hospitalization in a university hospital. He was treated conventionally and released on combination insulin therapy, with a total of 55 units a day. His other medical problems included 50% vision loss, thought to be a secondary complication of the diabetes, elevated serum prostate specific antigen (PSA) and extensive coronary artery disease documented by the presence of several significant circulation abnormalities (ischemia) by special stress-imaging testing.

Bio-resonance testing discovered systemic mercury intoxication of a dental origin, affecting many organs including the pancreas, coronary arteries and prostate gland. Several opportunistic infectious agents, especially *Candida albicans* and parasites, were present. These infections usually evolve in the background of metal-induced immune deficiency and disturbance of normal intestinal bacterial flora caused by antibiotics. Repeated blood testing confirmed the presence of mercury in his body.

Treatment: Primarily with homeopathic isodes and appropriate homeopathic and glandular organ support. In anticipation of recovery of his pancreatic and general metabolic functions, the patient was advised to begin tapering off his daily insulin dose gradually in order to avoid hypoglycemic attacks.

Follow-up: One month later, insulin therapy was discontinued and his blood sugar concentration was in the low normal range. Two months after homeopathic therapy was initiated and continued on a periodic basis, his vision was completely restored. Several months later, while continuing the homeopathic regimen, the patient upon his own request was placed on weekly intravenous infusions of EDTA chelation therapy to enhance the treatment of his atherosclerotic vascular disease. The previously elevated serum PSA concentration decreased four-fold and became normal. One year after the initial abnormal cardiac imaging scan, although the patient had not been placed on any strict low-fat diet, cholesterol-lowering agents, or heart medications, the doctor who evaluated the test concluded: *"I have compared this study to the previous study, and I do not see the findings previously reported. Based on my review, this study appears within normal limits. I see no definite evidence of ischemia or infarction."*

Three years later, in the November 28, 2002 issue of *The New England Journal of Medicine,* mercury was implicated as a serious causative factor in the development of cardiovascular disease.

A bizarre case

A teenager had suffered since birth with chronic fatigue, numerous food and environmental allergies, and bizarre spells consisting of sudden fainting, followed by assuming a fetal position, talking like a baby and hitting anyone around. He had been evaluated by many conventional specialists in a university hospital and was determined to be feigning and in need of psychiatric care. Treatments with alternative medicine and allergy desensitizations were unsuccessful. He remained unable to attend school and was home-schooled with difficulty due to physical and mental fatigue.

Bio-resonance testing revealed multiple endocrinopathies of potentially life-threatening nature along with multiple chronic viral, parasitic and fungal infections. The main culprit was chronic heavy metal toxicity with lead and mercury. These findings were then confirmed with conventional tests.

Treatment: He was treated primarily with homeopathic lead and mercury isodes combined with proper homeopathic and glandular organ support.

Follow-up: Conventional lab tests documented that both the lead and mercury could no longer be detected following the homeopathic treatment and the patient was able to make excellent progress in his health and schoolwork for several months until he discontinued his visits.

A case of reversed coronary artery disease

A 43-year-old man suffered from the chest pain, cold sweats and weakness typical of heart angina. Cardiac imaging stress testing yielded images consistent with a diagnosis of coronary artery occlusion.

Bio-resonance testing identified the presence of cadmium, silver amalgam and mercury in the coronary arteries and other organs.

Treatment: Homeopathic isodes of cadmium, silver amalgam and mercury were administered in proper potencies with the corresponding homeopathic organ support, along with short-term use of heart medication.

Follow-up: No chest pains were experienced, even after heart medications were discontinued. Several months later, the same stress test with cardiac imaging resulted in completely normal findings.

Note: No cholesterol-lowering drugs or low-fat diet were prescribed at any time.

A strange cystitis

A middle-aged celibate woman exhibited a very toxic general state, complaining of high fever, chills, and severe weakness. The symptoms had begun a few days previously when she had started experiencing severe discomfort and burning on urination and noticed a cloudy urine. She was seen in a nearby emergency room and placed on antibiotic therapy. However, her condition continued to deteriorate.

Bio-resonance testing identified a bacterial infection in the urinary bladder.

Treatment: A classical homeopathic remedy, based on her overall state, was administered.

Follow-up: Two days later, she reported 50% improvement and was given the next cycle of homeopathic therapy. However, after a few days, she reported only a minor improvement which was very unusual because in my experience, the great majority of infectious diseases normally respond very well to this approach and without the use of antibiotics. Therefore, a more serious pathology was suspected. Based upon the bacterial strain identified, a connection was suspected between the urogenital system and her gastrointestinal tract. As a result, her lower abdominal gastrointestinal organs became a particular focus of Bio-resonance testing. It suggested a very alarming finding—perforation of the lower colon and a fistula that had formed, exposing the urogenital tract to continuous contamination with colonic contents. When questioned, she admitted to having undergone several successive high colonic enemas which involved the delivery of large volumes of water under high pressure through a mechanical device. She was sent immediately to a nearby hospital to undergo an MRI scan in order to confirm the diagnosis. The scan did confirm the presence of the fistula detected by Bio-resonance testing. She had surgery on the same day, which saved her life.

A cured case of severe fibromyalgia and mysterious joint disease

An elderly man suffered from a great number of debilitating symptoms over several years. They consisted of excruciating joint and muscle pains that made even the slightest movements unbearable and obtaining any rest or sleep nearly impossible. In addition, he suffered from intense jerking and twitching of his muscles, impairment of peripheral vision, extreme swelling with intense heat, and redness of his legs and hands. He felt extremely cold and had symptoms of chronic fatigue syndrome. He was evaluated over the years by several rheumatologists at the local university hospital and underwent extensive lab and imaging tests which included x-rays, MRI and CAT scans of his chest, abdomen and pelvis. All of these revealed some non-specific abnormalities, including very high plasma concentration of *C-reactive protein,* indicative of the presence of a severe inflammatory process of unknown origin. According to the patient, *"They gave me 5 to 6 diagnoses, but none of them held up. Every week they gave me a new diagnosis and were going to place me on high-dose prednisone and anti-inflammatory drugs. I finally got tired of all this . . . and left."* The patient also undertook numerous alternative medical modalities, such as acupuncture, classical homeopathy, chiropractic, massage, herbal and nutritional supplementation and diet therapies. None were effective.

When he first appeared in my office, the most recent conventional diagnosis was that of severe fibromyalgia or some other undetermined disease. During this first visit, he appeared to be extremely debilitated, and was in so much pain that he could hardly rise off his chair or walk without help.

Bio-resonance testing identified systemic intoxication with mercury, particularly in his bone marrow and musculoskeletal system, and the presence of several parasitic agents and opportunistic fungal infections. A proper and primarily homeopathic treatment was instituted based on these findings.

Follow-up: In just his third visit, the patient asserted, "I'm just about cured, doctor." On the whole, about 90% of his symptoms were resolved and he was able to resume his usual daily activities, including workouts at the local YMCA. Overall, his quality of life was restored.

Further follow-up evaluations not only confirmed his cure but also his renewed health. In parallel with his clinical improvement, the plasma *C-reactive protein* concentration became normal.

Breast cancer reversed?

A middle-aged woman with a strong family history of breast cancer became alarmed after detecting a solid mass in her breast. An ultrasound examination of her breast confirmed the presence of a *solid mass demonstrating hypervascular flow.* ("Hypervascular flow" implies increased blood supply, which is a common hallmark of cancerous tumors because as they grow, they develop their own extensive vasculature.) *The finding is suspicious for malignancy.*

Her mammography report stated that: *"There is centimeter retroareolar mass with smooth margins, findings suspicious for malignancy. Please note supplemental sonogram demonstrates this mass to be solid, with intrinsic blood flow, findings compatible with malignancy."*

The patient was scheduled for surgery to remove her entire breast. While awaiting the surgery date, she underwent two homeopathic treatments, based on the findings of Bio-resonance testing. The following toxicological agents were detected in her tumorous breast: copper, osmium, mercury, gallium and cobalt. All of these agents were addressed with the corresponding homeopathic isodes, each administered in the potency indicated by the testing and followed by the appropriate homeopathic organ support. The testing also detected parasitic organisms in the same breast. A combination herb and medication treatment was prescribed.

Follow-up: Several days after completion of the treatment, the patient reported that she felt that her mass had diminished in size. Nevertheless, she proceeded with the plans for her scheduled mastectomy. As a matter of good medical practice, an initial biopsy sample of the area was obtained in order to ascertain the exact type of malignancy present and determine whether radiation or chemotherapy would be required. The pathological examination failed to find any evidence of malignancy and reported it as benign. The surgery was cancelled and the patient was discharged immediately. The surgeon confirmed that, based on the mammogram, the sonographic reports and his own physical examination prior to the biopsy, a cancerous tumor had indeed been present and had apparently undergone complete remission.

Severe cardiomyopathy reversed

A man in his fifties complained of weakness and shortness of breath, even during mild exertion. He had been diagnosed with severe impairment of his heart muscle (the myocardium). A nuclear imaging test had revealed extremely poor contractility. He also had a 25-year history of hypertension. Consequently, he was suffering from congestive heart failure and was taking high doses of diuretic and blood pressure medications.

Bio-resonance testing revealed the presence of cadmium and mercury in the myocardium.

Treatment: Homeopathic cadmium and mercury remedies with proper homeopathic organ support were administered. Homeopathic mercury in different potencies was repeated on two more occasions. Within the period of only a few months, the patient experienced complete clinical recovery and was able to return to his regular heavy physical work on a daily basis. His cardiac contractility increased four-and-a-half fold (from 10% to 45.5%, with the norm being 50%–70%), and all of his medications were discontinued. Neither his congestive heart failure nor hypertension ever returned.

When "cholesterol-lowering went bad"

A gentleman in his fifties consistently tested adversely to a cholesterol-lowering drug that had been prescribed by his allopathic doctor. Bio-resonance testing demonstrated that this drug was harming his liver. Each time he was advised to discontinue the drug, fear instilled by the cholesterol hysteria prevented him from following the recommendation. However, six months after the medication was started, he was taken by ambulance to a nearby hospital with excruciating pains in his liver. A blood test confirmed the presence of severe liver inflammation and he was advised by the hospital doctors to discontinue the cholesterol-lowering drug immediately.

A case of near-fatal heart arrhythmia

A man in his forties developed a life-threatening heart arrhythmia, ventricular tachycardia, following a massive heart attack. The arrhythmia was completely out of control despite several heart medications and he remained in extremely high risk of sudden death at any time. His cardiologist recommended that he undergo a sophisticated electrophysiologic heart study in the hospital in order to determine the most effective antiarrhythmic medication, but he refused.

Bio-resonance testing identified one of his heart medications as the trigger of the arrhythmia. After the drug was discontinued, the arrhythmia disappeared.

Chapter *7*

Bio-Resonance Testing—How Does it Work?

What are the mechanisms underlying Bio-resonance testing EAV and Applied Kinesiology? Physics has established that every substance is endowed with its own unique *natural (electromagnetic) resonance frequency.* Bio-resonance testing uses the ability of the body to sense the frequency field of a substance and respond accordingly.

The Taiwanese physicist Professor Kuo-Gen Chen concluded that the well-known phenomenon of resonance in physics is responsible for the communication between the organs and testing vials in EAV. He also asserted that homeopathic remedies work on the same resonance principle.[274]

Several mechanisms have been proposed to explain the phenomena of Applied Kinesiology testing:

* Ascending (afferent) neural pathways deliver sensory signals (heat, cold, pain, etc.) from the skin through the spinal cord to various brain centers, including those handling involuntary muscle reflexes. From there, a response appropriate to the significance of the incoming information—"alarm" or "no alarm"—is issued. This response is communicated to the peripheral muscle groups via the spinal cord and the motor nerves which activate the muscles.

* Professor Tiller believes that between the 600,000 miles of total nerve tissue contained in the body and acupuncture meridians, there is plenty of "wire" to serve as both receiving and transmitting antennas to deliver information to and from either end of the circuit. Such antennas could explain how humans are able to receive information from sources outside of their immediate physi-

cal contact. He also proposes that subtle energetic interactions between a tested substance and a patient's subconscious are transmitted via *subtle fields* and play an important role in kinesiological testing. This hypothesis presupposes that the subconscious or conscious brain contains all of the information that concerns any area or aspect of the body, including sick or stressed organs and the causes of illness.[275]

• Neurophysiological research has demonstrated that the continuous DC current flowing through perineural tissue between the skin and brain might represent a primary communication response system in our body. Named a *DC analog system,* it has been shown in experiments to become activated even before brain cells undergo the electrical activation that initiates a decision. It is of interest to note that perineural cells arise embryiologically from the same tissue, the *ectoderm,* that also gives rise to all skin and nerve cells. It is conceivable that the DC system might even be the primary command center of the central nervous system.[276]

• The hypothesis that the brain and its main stress control centers are involved in the phenomenon of Bio-resonance has been confirmed by observations that "the master gland"—the *hypothalamus*—is disturbed in cases involving disease or significant physical or emotional stress. After all, the hypothalamus is called "the master gland" because it regulates our endocrine system and is closely connected with immune and neuro-vegetative nervous systems as well as our emotions.

There is a growing body of evidence that the human brain and body function as a very sophisticated cybernetic unity where information is spread, shared and stored throughout its space-time boundaries in a holographic fashion. This implies that every cell in the body is informed about the state of the entire organism.[277–280] This hypothesis has gained considerable support recently from some puzzling observations that have followed organ transplant surgeries. Provocatively, the recipients of various organs (heart, kidney, liver and others) appear to have inherited many personality traits of their donors. In one extreme case, the recipient of an organ from the opposite gender experienced a change in sexual preference.[281]

Clinical Studies and Experience Concerning the Accuracy of Bio-Resonance Diagnosis

A number of studies have been performed worldwide:

• In a pilot study, Dr. Irmer of Germany, an associate of Dr. Voll, used EAV to diagnose 81 patients with chronic appendicitis. All of these patients were completely asymptomatic in the appendix area, which was considered to be very unusual because this condition is of an inflammatory nature and potentially life-threatening. Subsequent surgery confirmed the diagnosis in 100% of the cases.[282]

• In a small clinical study of 11 patients presented with different medical problems (infectious, neurological, gastrointestinal, and several different malignancies), the results of EAV agreed with those of standard diagnostic tests.[283]

• In a study of 120 subjects, a positive and statistically significant correlation was found between the EAV findings and blood test results that indicated that pesticides were present in the body.[284]

• Several studies concerning diabetes and hypertension confirmed the ability of EAV diagnosis to detect problems in the internal organs that are involved in these illnesses.[285–288]

• In a study conducted at the UCLA School of Medicine in Los Angeles, thirty individuals were tested "blindly" with EAV. Four lung cancer patients were "mixed" with 26 subjects who had negative chest x-rays and were considered to be healthy by conventional criteria. The four cancer patients were identified correctly. Of the 26 subjects with negative chest x-rays, 22 were deemed by EAV to have normal respiratory systems. However, EAV discovered four cases of previously unsuspected respiratory problems. This outcome is consistent with the experience of skilled practitioners of Bio-resonance testing, who often detect cellular energetic changes in tissues years before conventional clinical tests are able to reveal organ pathology. Most conventional tests are fairly insensitive at these early stages and able to detect only full-blown disease.[289]

• E. Hoellischer, MD, of Germany conducted a study on patients with heart disease, using a sophisticated analysis of their heart images obtained with infrared thermography. During imaging, the patients held a glass-sealed homeopathic remedy that had been deemed effective in the treatment of their conditions by favorable EAV measurements of heart meridian acupuncture points. After 15 minutes in each case, thermographic images reflecting improvement in cardiac function were recorded. At the same time, the EAV measurements of the previously "sick" points began to improve, too. Furthermore, after 15 minutes of being held, the injection of the same homeopathic remedies into the "sick" points produced only very modest additional improvement, suggesting that these hand-held remedies had already triggered healing to the extent that further stimulation with injection of the same remedies could not add much of a "push".[290]

Dr. Hoellischer's experience is reminiscent of a very interesting case I encountered some years ago in my practice, confirming the energy-field mode of action on the part of homeopathic remedies:

A Christian priest in his 60's complained of intense chest pains. He had been experiencing them for three months following a serious heart attack. "It is like a wound in my heart, doctor. It is there day and night, and even when I am asleep, I feel it." Various medications prescribed by his cardiologists failed to afford any relief. He was told that the medications were ineffective because his coronary arteries were badly blocked, as evidenced by cardiac catheterization. Bypass surgery was inevitable and considered urgent in order to save his life. His prognosis looked grim. The fear of surgery was too great, however, to allow him to agree to the operation. This pot-bellied, benevolent man made it very clear that he could not relate either to a strict diet or to alternative medicine generally and even less to homeopathy in particular. He was a bit wary of what he called my "very strange homeopathic questions," but out of kindness, he provided me with short and vague answers. As a result, I was not at all sure what the correct classical homeopathic remedy would be to match his specific complaints and so decided to use Bio-resonance testing to assess several remedies that could be helpful.

While I was preparing the remedies for testing, I heard a loud snoring from the direction of the examining table and found the good priest to be in a deep sleep. I describe these facts preceding the testing to make it clear that neither the patient (whose sleep indicated a lack of interest) nor the doctor (in a state of uncertainty) created a situation that was in any way conducive to producing a placebo effect.

I placed in his hand a metal bar, connected via a cable, to a testing platform and began the testing. His "first most stressed organ", not surprisingly, was determined to be the coronary arteries. I left the coronary artery vial on the platform and proceeded matching it against the remedies I had chosen, placing these, one at a time, on a testing platform without looking at them. The third remedy in the sequence demonstrated its effectiveness by triggering a favorable muscle reflex response. I placed it aside and was reaching out for the next one when my good patient suddenly stopped snoring, opened his eyes and asked what was in that tube that I had just used. "My chest pain, doctor, for some reason, as of a few seconds ago, has just suddenly stopped." I looked up at the vial that I just set aside—it was Latrodectus Mactans *in 12X, one of the best homeopathic remedies for heart attacks accompanied with intense pain and a sensation of deep injury to the heart.*

Having realized that the remedy "took" and had already begun its therapeutic action, I stopped further testing and advised the patient to take the remedy home but refrain from repeating its use unless the pain returned. I made it clear to him that it was impossible to know how long the therapeutic action would last—minutes, days, or weeks and asked him to let me know when and if he needed to administer the remedy again. Three weeks later he reported that he was completely free of chest pain for 14 days following the testing. When it returned, it had barely 20% of the intensity of the original pain. He had then placed 1 pellet of the remedy into his mouth and the pain left him for good. I followed him for over a year, until he moved out of the area. The remedy never had to be repeated.

In this regard, I might also add that in many cases, I have had patients tell me during testing that they felt some unpleasant sensations in their sick organs while, unbeknownst to them, they were being subjected to the field of the very organs through the corresponding homeopathic vials.

* In a blind study conducted with Applied Kinesiology testing, a greater than 90% positive correlation was found between food allergies identified with this method and the patients' immunological "food allergy blood profile."[291]
* Applied Kinesiology testing provided very accurate assessments when study subjects were issuing true or false statements about themselves.[292] The involuntary reflex response assessed by AK in this case is based upon the same premise as are biofeedback and polygraph lie detector tests.[293,294]

The screening security tests recently adopted by law enforcement agencies at airports is based upon the similar autonomic reflex response. It monitors a person's simple iris response, using a special device during interrogation that differentiates true from false statements. Applied Kinesiology testing, especially the "non-force" method I use, has unlimited potential to assess veracity without relying upon specialized equipment.

Some physiologic studies have confirmed the mind-soma connection by registering the changes in electrical activity in muscles that occur in response to emotional stimuli, using electromyography instrumentation.[295]

Nationally acclaimed American psychiatrist David R. Hawkins, MD, PhD, who has been using Applied Kinesiology testing extensively in his work, reported unfailing 100% reliability during a fifteen-year study conducted by alternative medicine psychiatrist John Diamond, MD, and his associates. In this study, complete correlation was observed between positive and negative emotional and mental attitudes and the intensity of involuntary muscle responses. Weak responses, which invariably occurred while a person was issuing a false statement, were accompanied by desynchronization of the electrical activity of the cerebral hemispheres.[296,297]

It is noteworthy to mention that the U.S. Patent Office issued several patents for medical diagnosis on behalf of Applied Kinesiology and EAV, thereby acknowledging the scientific validity of Bio-resonance diagnosis.

Chapter 8

Homeopathic Vaccines and Antidotes. Can They be Mass Produced Faster and More Cheaply than Conventional Vaccines?

It takes years to test and produce a conventional anti-viral or anti-bacterial vaccine. Even then, the mass demand may not be met on short notice. An anthrax vaccine, for example, is still not available for public use. Furthermore, vaccines or drugs that would render increased resistance to the deleterious health effects of chemical or nuclear warfare or enhance detoxification virtually do not exist. Here, homeopathically prepared antidotes and vaccines offer considerable advantage in ease, cost and speed of production.

Information frequencies can be reproduced electronically like CD's, amplified and imprinted into plain water media within seconds. Water impregnated with these frequencies will thereby represent an electronically cloned homeopathic remedy that is capable of eliciting the same physiologic response as the hand-prepared remedy.

Numerous experiments conducted by European researchers have confirmed unequivocally that electronic cloning of homeopathic remedies is feasible and clinically effective. These experiments involved active physiological, biological or toxicological substances (histamines, hormones, bacterial toxins, carcinogenic chemicals and others), transferred electronically through simple equipment into sealed water vials. Digitally made remedies were tested blindly, without the researchers knowing whether they were transferring an active substance or placebo into water media. Some experiments were repeated dozens of times and yielded consistently positive results.[298–304] In one experiment, the frequency of a homeopathic hormonal preparation was recorded on a CD which was then scanned into water. The original homeopathic hormonal substance and the one that was created by scanning into water from the

CD had comparable physiologic effects on lab animals. This experiment was performed blindly. Results compared favorably against the effects of treatment with a placebo.[305]

The principle of digital transference of information frequencies has been known in physics for decades. It was implemented in the early 1970's by scientists in the former West Germany. For example, F. Morrell, MD, and the electronic engineer, E. Rasche, built a bio-electronic instrument, MORA—an EAV diagnostic device that also contained a unit that can make any remedy in any desired potency upon the turn of a dial. This has enabled physicians to produce homeopathic remedies within one to two minutes, including poisonous and infectious agents and patients' own toxic or infected body fluids and discharges. This unit also is capable of reproducing and transferring already prepared remedies into water, suggesting the capability of reproducing remedies indefinitely. Some other European companies have been able to produce non-diagnostic remedy-making units with a substantial reduction in remedy production time. These compact and lightweight digital transfer units are compact—the size of a medium-sized jewelry box, and are not dependent on any external power source, using built-in magnetic energy. German physicist, Professor Wolfgang Ludwig, in his hundred-page report, *Biophysical Diagnosis and Therapy in the Ultrafine Energy Range,* confirmed the scientific validity of the homeopathic digital aspects of MORA and similar devices and expressed full confidence that once the basic principles of physics were allowed by mainstream medicine in everyday practice, *digital homeopathy* would open vast medical frontiers.

Tens of thousands of physicians in Europe use these devices successfully to prepare good quality homeopathic remedies from patients' own body fluids and to convert harmful substances of any kind into healing frequencies. These units can be indispensable; they can be used right in the midst of a biological, chemical or nuclear disaster to save countless lives by enabling homeopathic antidotes to be prepared and administered very rapidly. If built and utilized for mass production, these units would be able to produce hundreds of thousands of homeopathic digital antidotes in a single day.

One caveat: There are some companies that produce EAV computerized devices and claim that numerous remedies recorded into hard-drive discs can be extracted at any time without a compromise in quality. These companies, as a rule, have not used actual homeopathic remedies for inscription into the discs but rather their inexact surrogates. In my experience, these products are of inferior quality.

If afforded with the right technology, without a doubt, digital homeopathy holds tremendous potential for providing timely medical help to civilians and the military.

Chapter 9

How You Can Help to Protect Yourself and Your Family in Case of Biological, Chemical, or Nuclear Warfare

Water is a perfect receiver of information, thanks to its physico-chemical properties. It can be used first to absorb any harmful elements, biological, chemical or nuclear, from the contaminated environment, food or water supplies, bodily fluids or discharges. They can then be converted into energetic forms of homeopathic vaccine-antidotes.

Homeopathic remedies have been prepared from imponderant matter such as x-rays or sun and moon rays. This is not "mystic science" as the scientifically-illiterate would portray homeopathy. Water is capable of absorbing information from various forms of radiation, including those, as just mentioned, that are known to produce leukemia and melanomas or to trigger convulsions in epileptics.

The Method of Preparation of Isodes When the Toxic or Biological Agents are in the Environment

Examples: The World Trade Center dust and smoke fumes following September 11, anthrax or other biological agents (viral, bacterial, fungal) in the internal ventilation system of buildings, or the accidental or deliberate release of toxic gases or nuclear materials.

Accessories Needed

1. One half-ounce or one-ounce dropper bottles—available from a local pharmacy or medical-surgical supply store.

   In the event that you are caught by surprise and the recommended dropper bottles are not available, you may use any glass or even hard plastic containers. These might be bottles from sodas or jars from tomato sauce, etc., as long as they have a screw top and are thoroughly cleaned with scalding hot water and rinsed with cold water.

2. Water
    * Filtered water from a well or from your town water supply (see NOTE on bottled spring water below).
    * Avoid distilled water unless you are extremely allergic and cannot tolerate any other water. Its energetic value is very low compared to natural clean water.
    * Your bottle should be filled with cold water to approximately ¾ of its volume. Do not use hot or warm water. Room temperature and refrigerated water are your second and third best choices, correspondingly.
    * Keep stored water away from EMF-emitting devices—computers, TV, ovens, etc.—or direct lighting, particularly fluorescent light which contains and energetically emits mercury, one of the most potent poisons on earth.

NOTE: Spring water is not necessarily superior in purity to filtered tap water, since industrial contamination or EPA violations may take place within the vicinities of the spring water source. A recently published survey found that town water samples on average were superior to spring waters. Contamination may sometimes take place only if temporarily.

Not long ago, several of my patients became ill seemingly for no particular reason. Through Bio-resonance testing, it was determined that a particular toxic metal was the culprit. It was quite puzzling because many of these patients came from diverse geographical areas. After collecting careful environmental and dietary histories, it turned out that all of them were consuming the same famous brand of spring water. All of these patients produced a stressful muscle reflex response while holding that brand in their hand, thus pointing it out as being the source of their illness. All of them promptly recovered after the isode of that metal was administered. When Bio-resonance testing was repeated some months later, new bottles of the same brand were found to be benign. Afterwards, some of these patients undertook,

*through the internet, a thorough study of environmental con-
ditions in the state where the spring water had come from.
Eventually they discovered that there was a chemical manufacturer in the area who had been caught and heavily pe-
nalized by the EPA for dumping toxic wastes into state water resources. By no coincidence, these wastes contained the
very metal that was detected by Bio-resonance testing. The
company could not meet the heavy burden of the penalties,
went bankrupt and ceased operation. The water company
seemed to have known about a possible contamination of
their product, because when confronted by some of these patients, it rushed to recall dispensers, including all of the water supplies, and promptly returned money and released
contracts.*

Preparation

1. Fill the bottle approximately ½ full.
2. To collect an air sample, remove the dropper and squeeze fully, making sure that no aspirated water is left inside. Place a bottle in the contaminated area. Depending upon how heavily contaminated the environment is or how urgently one needs to administer the remedy, the vessel may remain exposed to the air from a few minutes to several hours. On average, 20-30 minutes is ample time to allow the water to absorb the necessary elements. Another way to increase the absorbent surface of water would be to leave it exposed to the external environment if only for several minutes, in a cup or a bowl. Its contents can be poured into an empty bottle. Again, place it away from computers, faxes, TV, phones and direct fluorescent light.
3. Screw the dropper back on tightly so as not to allow any leakage. To save time and spare yourself the necessity of having a row of bottles graduated in potency to the desired strength, you can use a simplified preparation method known as *Korsakov's method,* named after General S.N. Korsakov, a personal homeopath of the Russian Tsar Nicholas I. This method has been accepted as legitimate by homeopathic pharmacists.
4. After you have made sure that the bottle is closed tightly, strike

the bottom of the bottle a dozen times. Any object that is hard enough and will not risk breaking the bottle will suffice: a thick or hardcover book, piece of carpet, even your hand, will work. Or, you may choose to shake the bottle vigorously a dozen times in a vertical position, provided it is not completely filled.

5. Remove the dropper and squeeze again. Pour the *entire* contents of the bottle out and discard it. Each time you do this, try, if possible, to avoid coming in contact with the water you are discarding; otherwise it will begin interacting through your skin before you have prepared a desired potency. You may wish to wear latex gloves.

Remember: Each time you replace the dropper, make sure you do not squeeze the dropper accidentally, which would allow the contents to aspirate automatically before a desired potency has been achieved.

6. Fill the bottle again approximately ¾ full.

Do ***not*** be overly concerned about following these instructions perfectly:

◆ The level to which you fill the bottle is exactly the same and fixed. In an emergency, it will not matter whether your measurements are exact as long as the bottle is not completely filled.

◆ You have discarded your entire solution. There always are a few residual drops remaining on the bottle walls. That is more than sufficient to assure a continuous transfer of information. Put the pharmaceutical mass-oriented mindset aside and think of a tiny drop as a microchip that emits signals in frequencies. These will instantly recharge the new portion of water that you add each time and/or as soon as you deliver even a few impacts or shake it well.

Each cycle of preparation increases the potency of your remedy by a strength of 1K, where K stands for Korsakov's potency. Six cycles will yield 6K potency, 12 cycles will yield 12K potency, and so on.

◆ Occasionally, you may lose your impact count. It may turn out to be one or two more, or less—this will not matter that much. It would be advisable, however, to keep a written count of the cycles and have a table handy with numbers from 1 to 100 or more available where you can quickly mark off each cycle.

Keep in mind that this principle of obtaining a contaminated sample can be applied to anything which bears traces of toxic agents: clothing, shoes, skin, hair, etc. Under these circumstances, one can simply swab the contaminated surface with a wet cotton swab or gauze and then by immersing or squeezing one of them briefly into a dropper bottle, it will deliver the sufficient amount of the toxin to prepare a homeopathic vaccine-antidote. In order to protect your hands when squeezing potentially contaminated gauze, you would be advised to wear impermeable gloves. If you wish to reuse the bottle that contained a prepared homeopathic remedy, you must irrigate the bottle and the eye-dropper with scalding water.

Approximate Guidelines for Selecting the Homeopathic Potencies to Use

NOTE: Before undertaking homeopathic treatment, it is very important to be thoroughly familiar with the potential blocks and draining factors presented in Chapter 13, under *General Environmental and Toxic Factors*. These factors might seriously impair treatment.

Potency choice—the higher the potencies, the more stimulating the remedy will be. The rule, "the more the better," does not apply here. Elderly persons or those who have been seriously weakened—to begin with or by the assault itself—may not mount enough energy to meet the demand of higher potencies. They would be better served by starting at the lower range: 6K, 9K or 12K. I would recommend applying the same criteria to people who have overactive immune systems, such as patients with autoimmune disorders, or a known history of multiple environmental and food allergies. In these individuals, the initial potency may be limited to 3K. A similar caution must be exercised with immuno-compromised people with AIDS, chemo- or radiation-therapy patients, people who suffer from chronic diseases, and those who take immuno-suppressive drugs such as prednisone or chemotherapeutic agents. The initial starting potency for them would be 6K, not to exceed 9K. One can always increase the potency later, if necessary. People with stronger constitutions can tolerate potencies of 15K, 30K, or up to 400K from the start.

What potency would one prefer to start with? A rule of thumb is, the higher the level of contamination or the more pronounced the symptoms, the higher the potency needed to mitigate the illness.

For *children,* the initial potencies are graduated:
• up to 3 years of age—6K—9K
• 3–10 years of age—12K
• older than 10 years—use the same general criteria that was used for adults

For **average adults,** the potencies are higher:
• mild cases—9K or 12K
• moderate cases—15K—30K
• severe cases—60K—90K
• very severe cases—150K—200K—400K

The first three categories will constitute the majority.

It undoubtedly would be far less time-consuming, particularly in cases of high potencies, if the Food and Drug Administration (FDA) would approve portable potency making devices for mass use.

Quantity: One drop of any of the potencies, placed under the tongue, is sufficient. In cases where a person or small child cannot cooperate, several drops can be squeezed quickly into the mouth. If this is difficult, for whatever reasons, one may choose to place a few drops on either a pacifier or a piece of favorite food. Do not allow someone to drink large quantities of liquid, more than a sip or two, if a remedy was placed in it. Otherwise this may lead to overstimulation.

It is a good idea to have on hand at least a dozen spare empty bottles, stocking labels, and an extra supply of clean water. There is, after all, a hypothetical risk that water reservoirs may be targeted for contamination. As you proceed with the potency making, place a few drops of lower potencies (3K or 6K) into separate bottles before you go to higher potencies. Fill these bottles ¾ full and shake them vigorously to assure a proper admixture. Label them correspondingly, i.e., 3K or 6K, add the date and identify a suspected contamination source (i.e., anthrax, smallpox, air dust, toxic gas or nuclear radiation, etc.). There are several reasons for saving these: one, you may need them at a later time, several days or even weeks later after the higher potencies have run their course; two, progress may have been achieved but some mild residual symptoms may still linger, possibly due to some residual contamination or infection remaining in the environment; three, children or elderly or debilitated adults may need lower potencies. Should you save these bottles, simply borrow a few drops from the corresponding bottle, place them into another bottle, fill it up ¾ of the volume and go up to your next higher potency following the preparation process.

In cases of nuclear contamination in the air or the consumption of radioactive water supplies, the initial potency of a remedy prepared in either instance should be at least 30K and should be administered 2–3 times a day for the length of exposure.

Note: Before repeating a remedy of the same potency, deliver a few hard impacts against the bottom of its container. This will increase its strength somewhat and will help prevent the development of resistance to the same potency.

How to proceed after an initial remedy is consumed

Remember, it is not possible to render exhaustive and rigid guidelines beforehand. These guidelines are designed to minimize the initial damage in an emergency before qualified medical help becomes available. When help arrives, further services will be provided by health care professionals who, it is to be hoped, will be properly trained in homeopathy and Bio-resonance testing.

Before we consider general guidelines, you need to keep in mind that unlike pharmaceutical substances, which exert action only for as long as they are repeated, usually in short intervals, homeopathic remedies act by jump-starting your own healing process and allowing your body to do the rest. Therefore, if one dose is sufficient to provide a strong enough "turn on" signal and your body is able to mobilize sufficient reserves to overcome completely an offending agent, the first dose may be curative.

On the other hand, if only partial relief has been achieved and progress has ceased, a repeat dose may be necessary.

Several potential scenarios should be considered before proceeding further:

1. You took the remedy, one drop, and there was no improvement within 2 hours: Double the potency, i.e., from 3K to 6K, or from 6K to 12K, etc., and repeat dosing. If there still is no effect after

two more hours, which would be very unlikely, double the potency.

2. Improvement follows the initial dosing and symptoms gradually disappear or continue to regress: No further action is necessary. Wait!

   If the potential for recontamination exists, you may repeat the same potency every 3–4 days until such a threat becomes remote.

3. Improvement lasts for 6–8 hours or a day or two, but some residual symptoms persist or the symptoms return: Repeat the same potency and wait 2 more hours. One of several potential outcomes will most likely occur:

   * Healing progresses: No further immediate action is necessary.
   * Fairly good positive response results in better progress than the original initial dose but symptoms persist and progress ceases: Repeat the same potency again.
   * Only mild response occurs with no better result than the initial dosing: Double the potency and administer a drop.

   Follow these same general principles in assessing your further responses and action.

4. In the unlikely case of complete absence of clinical response, suspect the presence of blocks and draining factors (see Chapter 13 under *General Environmental and Toxic Factors*). If these are ruled out and qualified medical help is unavailable, move to therapy with autoisopathics described in the section, *"Treatment With Your Own Body Fluids—Homeopathic Autoisopathy for Biological and Toxic Assaults."*

Summary of Precautions

Be sure to remember these specific instructions:

* Avoid distilled water unless it is the only source of uncontaminated water.
* Do not use hot or warm water.
* Keep homeopathic remedies, whether commercially prepared or made yourself, away from EMF-emitting devices or appliances (computers, TV, phones, faxes, direct sun and electric lighting, particularly fluorescent light, and magnets). The best environ-

ment in which to store remedies are closed cabinets or drawers. Avoid temperatures above 100°F. Apply the same precautions to stored water.

- Make sure no aspirated water is left inside the dropper in the course of preparation.
- Avoid touching the dropper or the remedy.

What Are the Signs of Improvement?

For a treatment to be deemed successful, do not expect every sign and symptom to improve or go away rapidly. The further the disease has progressed prior to treatment, the weaker the person may be and the slower the recovery. The most important criterion to monitor one's progress is the *energy* level of the person being treated. It is not only the matter of a subjective sense of better well-being but also a fundamental necessity for one's existence, for without proper energy level the organism is unable to carry out its physiologic functions and will cease to exist. Physics teaches us that even inanimate objects disintegrate unless they are endowed with sufficient energy to hold them together.

Signs that the energy-vitality state of a person has improved

Surplus energy will play a decisive role in the promotion of further healing. This can be assessed best through a comparison with baseline symptoms.

In general, these are the signs to look for in judging progress:

- overall, less "sickly" appearance
- decrease in pallor or excessive redness of the skin and face
- stronger voice
- better and clearer speech and thinking
- stronger and better-controlled body movements
- re-establishment of appetite and thirst
- desire to increase one's physical activity
- increased interest in social or family-related matters
- smiling
- change in perspiration pattern accompanied with an increase sense of well-being, i.e., excessive perspiration decreased or hot, dry skin began to perspire while fever was resolving
- re-establishment or improvement of normal elimination patterns

It is possible, though, that when the therapeutic response is positive, fever or perspiration may increase temporarily, referred to in homeopathy as a "healing crisis." This may occur because any homeopathic remedy (classical, isode or autoisode) may provoke the immune system to "go on the offensive." As a result, more dead viral and bacterial fragments enter the circulation (particularly in cases where biological agents are involved), temporarily irritating the thermo-regulation center of the brain. If this has happened following the use of an isode or autoisode remedy, proceed with lymphatic drainage by administering the remedy, *"Lymph-S,"* as soon as the body temperature begins to increase, and hydrate with water. If fever follows the administration of a classical homeopathic remedy, do not give *"Lymph-S"* or complex homeopathic remedies, but do assure proper hydration. If the rise in temperature heralds a healing crisis, it is usually short-lasting and will end in an hour or two, as the general state and well-being improve.

If a high fever, 103°F or higher, persists, and you do not have proper training in homeopathy or are not in possession of a good and detailed homeopathic first aid kit, use regular over-the-counter medications such as Tylenol or aspirin to reduce it, provided they are not contraindicated. Avoid aspirin in case of nuclear irradiation, as it may worsen the already potentially compromised tendency toward bleeding.

Signs that the most troubling energy-draining symptom has improved

This might be any symptom, such as high fever, intense chills, pain, difficulty breathing, persistent diarrhea or severe nausea.

As a rule, an increase in energy level and decrease in energy-draining symptoms occur together. If the patient improves following treatment, in all likelihood a breaking point in a disease process has been achieved.

Do not be dismayed if in the process of improvement or shortly preceding the appearance of improvement a new set of discharges appears through the sinuses, mouth, skin, bowels, or urogenital tract. Homeopathic remedies help the body to expel toxins through any body orifice and through the skin. The cardinal sign between these discharges, heralding healing or deterioration, would be a positive change in the overall general state.

A special note on recognizing and treating nuclear radiation

There are two major routes of entry of the ionizing radiation into the body, external and internal.

The external route includes nuclear weapons, nuclear plants, and medical treatments. Internal entry occurs by way of contaminated food and water supplies.[306]

Any organ can be affected by nuclear radiation, but the bone marrow and the thyroid gland are particularly vulnerable.

Due to the involvement of the bone marrow, which is the key blood and immune organ, as well as other important immune organs, thymus and spleen, the radiation illness sets forth a succession of immune and hematological dysfunctions.

The complete picture may vary greatly, depending upon the route, intensity, and length of exposure. Symptoms may include nausea and vomiting due to generalized toxicity. A drop in total blood and white counts may result in severe weakness, pallor, secondary infections, enlarged lymph nodes and bleeding. Hair loss is often a result of affected thyroid gland. Skin burns can be present. Depending upon the intensity and proximity to the external exposure site, skin symptoms may also ensue in the form of burns, blisters or ulcerations. Bad coughs may occur due to inhalation. Bloody diarrhea may result if contaminated food or water have been ingested.

A radiation illness should be suspected if inexplicable weakness, nausea, vomiting, skin burning, hair loss, or tendency to bruise or bleed appear and persist. Likewise, unexplained recurrence or development of persistent infections (e.g. herpes, sinusitis, bronchitis, cystitis, etc.) in the presence of these symptoms should alert you to a possibility of radiation exposure.

Conventional diagnostic methods consisting of examining swabs off skin, respiratory airways, rectum, blood counts, or 24-hour urine or even stool collection, are helpful in establishing the diagnosis. With the Bio-resonance testing, a diagnosis can be ascertained within seconds.

It is well-known that radiation causes cancer and leukemia which ensue over the years. Children of preadolescent age are particularly susceptible for two major reasons. Iodine absorption by the thyroid gland is increased in children for use in the production of thyroid hormone. This includes radioactive iodine found in nuclear power plants. Also in children, blood supply to the developing bone marrow is increased and this enhances the delivery of radiation poisons that lead to leukemia, anemia and other serious blood disorders. As the Chernobyl experience demonstrated, thyroid cancers became rampant among other malignancies in children following this disaster.

Strictly speaking, any tissue or organ is vulnerable depending on the degree of exposure and the pre-existing constitutional or genetic weaknesses. As an example, people who smoke or face occupational or urban exposures to pollution will have higher possibilities of pre-existing impairment in the respiratory system. Persons who have undergone recent or frequent mammographies, x-rays or CAT scan examinations will be at a higher risk to develop disease in the corresponding, pre-exposed part. For these reasons, it has been the author's experience that for best results, after the isodes have been administered, homeopathic support of weak organs, with organ preparations, *sarcodes,* should be given. This is to facilitate a release of the noxious elements by these organs and also to strengthen them. Even in the absence of Bio-resonance testing, a general sarcode formula inclusive of several key organs would be quite capable of playing a positive role.

In case of mild exposure to ionizing radiation, the recommended starting dose of nuclear isode for an adult is 12K, and for children, 30K. For a medium exposure—adults, 30K-60K; for children, 60K-90K. For severe exposure—both children and adults, 200K.

In either case, both the isode and sarcode formulas should be repeated at intervals ranging from once daily to once weekly, depending upon the severity and persistence of exposure and signs of radiation illness. As a general rule, it is better to administer these remedies more often than less often. This particularly applies to the sarcode formulas. On the average, lower potencies of radiation isode, 12K and 30K, should be followed an hour later with the sarcode formula. Higher potencies of isode, 60K-90K, should be followed by a sarcode formula in two hours; and 200K or higher isode potencies should be followed by a sarcode formula in three hours. The reason for this is that higher potencies work deeper in the body and are usually administered when the degree of intoxication is correspondingly deep. Therefore, they require a longer period of time to exert therapeutic action before sending the body the next "command" with a follow-through remedy.

In addition to homeopathic remedies, a good quality antioxidant formula administered three to four times a day would be appropriate. However, supplementation with the nutrients C, E, or garlic should not be excessive, as they are known to exert suppressive aspirin-like effects on the adhesiveness of blood platelets, which might be decreased already due to irradiation. Vitamins E and C should not exceed approximately 400 units or 1,000 mg a day correspondingly, and garlic pills should be restricted to one daily. Likewise, aspirin and other medications or supplements, such as fish oil or flaxseed oil, which exert similar action, should be withheld for the time.

Administration of the amino acid Lysine, 750mg, three-four times a day, would be helpful for people who suffer from flare-ups of herpes infection, which can be very painful. At least two capsules a day of good quality probiotic formula would be advisable, too, in order to contain opportunistic Candida yeast infections that intensify under conditions of immune suppression.

A few words about potassium iodide

Potassium iodide is recommended for protection of the thyroid gland only. In cases involving nuclear plants that contain radioactive iodine, known to be absorbed by a thyroid gland "hungry" for iodine, potassium iodide holds its therapeutic value only within the first 24 hours following the exposure and becomes ineffective thereafter. Consuming it prophylactically can be harmful, as it may cause a thyroid dysfunction.

Potassium iodide should be administered daily for as long as the exposure continues. The tablets distributed by our Federal agencies to states with nuclear plants are 130mg each—the daily dose for an average adult of 18 years of age and over. Children's dosages are specified below.[307] Keep in mind that this medicine is very salty and many children and infants will dislike the taste or be unable to swallow it. For this reason, it is recommended that the tablets be ground and dissolved in water first and disguised in drinks.

The FDA recommends several liquids to mitigate the taste (raspberry syrup in particular):

- raspberry syrup
- water
- low fat white milk
- low fat chocolate milk
- orange juice
- flat soda (cola, etc.)

You may also use baby formula, protein formula, or your child's favorite juice or drink.

Supplies and Preparation for Potassium Iodide solution
- Potassium iodide (KI) 130 mg tablet
- Metal teaspoon
- Small bowl
- The drink of your choice

1. **Grinding the potassium iodide tablet into powder**
    Put one 130mg potassium iodide tablet into a small bowl and grind it into a fine powder, using the back of the metal teaspoon against the inside of the bowl. The powder should not have any large pieces.
2. **Mixing potassium iodide powder into a drink**
    Add four teaspoonfuls of water to the potassium iodide powder in the small bowl. Use a spoon to mix them together until the potassium iodide powder has dissolved.
3. **Mix drink of choice with potassium iodide powder and water solution**
    Add four teaspoonfuls of drink to the potassium iodide powder and water mixture described in Step 2.

The amount of potassium iodide in the drink is 16.25mg per teaspoon. The number of teaspoonfuls to give your child depends upon your child's age. The potassium iodide in most of the drinks will keep for up to seven days in the refrigerator. The FDA recommends that the potassium iodide drink mixtures be prepared weekly. Unused portions should be discarded.

Daily dosages recommended for **infants and children** are as follows:

If your child is:	Give your child this amount of Potassium Iodide (KI)*	Which is
An adolescent between 12 and 18 years old*	**4 teaspoonfuls** or ½ tablet of 130mg tablet	65 mg of potassium iodide (KI)
Between 4 and 12 years old	**4 teaspoonfuls** or ½ tablet of 130mg tablet	65 mg of potassium iodide (KI)
Over 1 month through 3 years	**2 teaspoonfuls**	32.5 mg of potassium iodide (KI)
An infant from birth through 1 month	**1 teaspoonful**	16.25 mg of potassium iodide (KI)

*Adolescents approaching adult size [equal to or greater than 154 pounds (70 kg)] should receive the full adult dose (130 mg tablet or 8 teaspoonfuls of KI mixture).

Consult your physician or a pediatrician ahead of time concerning these dosages because they may vary according to individual medical history, state of health, pregnancy, lactation or other factors.

Should these measures become necessary, stay tuned into public health announcements. Be sure to contact your doctor or local hospital regarding any possible variations in the dosage or length of time to administer Potassium Iodide.

Clinical Examples of the Treatment of Toxicological, Biological and Nuclear Agents with Homeopathic Isodes

A case of industrial pollutants

A man in his 40's complained of chest pain that occurred at the end of each workday and was caused by heavy exposure to industrial pollutants. He was advised to leave an open one-ounce dropper bottle filled with water in his work area for 30–60 minutes and to bring it to my office, where an isode was prepared from this water, in several potencies. Using Bio-resonance testing, the 6K potency was determined to be the most effective and he was to take one drop at the end of each work day. The chest pains ceased within a few days. He continued this regimen for a year and a half and then stopped using it altogether. For more than two years, he has remained free of chest pain.

Comment: The homeopathic remedy not only assured prompt relief but also resulted in the development of long-term toxicological resistance.

A case of severe dermatitis

Following contact with a photographic fluid, a 14-year-old girl developed severe dermatitis on her hands with symptoms that included intense itching, redness and pain, and with oozing of thick glue-like discharge. Her face also was affected because she touched it when her hands were still wet with the fluid. Photographic fluid isode in 12K potency rapidly cleared her skin.

A case of narcolepsy

A woman in her 70's complained of unusual sleepiness during the daytime over a period of several months. She was concerned that she might fall asleep at the wheel of her car. Her physician could not find any apparent reason for her complaints. She was not taking any medications to account for side-effects.

Bio-resonance testing, nevertheless, revealed a pharmaceutical substance, belonging to the category of tranquilizers, in her brain. When questioned, she admitted to taking some kind of a sleeping pill intermittently in the past, the exact name of which she could not recall.

Treatment: complex homeopathic isode of a mixture of pharmaceutical tranquilizers, sleeping drugs, in 30X potency, one drop.

Follow-up: For 8 years since, she has never encountered another episode of narcolepsy.

A case of toxic fumigation

A young woman with multiple chemical sensitivities suffered from the toxic pest control fumigation conducted in her building on a weekly basis. She reacted with severe headaches, fatigue, anxiety and other debilitating symptoms. She was advised to leave an open ½ ounce water bottle outside of her apartment door at the time of fumigation. After fumigation was complete, she prepared and began taking fumigation isode in 12K potency, immediately before or after fumigation. This regimen ended her weekly suffering.

A case of severe hay fever

A middle-aged woman complained of severe hay fever symptoms that recurred every season for years. She complained of intense sneezing, sinus congestion with copious discharges and a low energy level. Nonprescription allergy drugs usually caused unacceptable side effects and a combination *"Hay Fever"* homeopathic remedy did not afford any relief. She was advised to leave an open half-ounce dropper bottle filled with water outside for an hour. After she began taking the prepared isode, one drop as needed for each attack, her hay fever abated.

A case of toxic alcohol consumption

A two-year old boy ingested 70% rubbing alcohol. Seconds later, he was rolling on the floor and screaming in pain. The worst case scenario of this situation was a potentially life-threatening perforation of the esophagus. Liver damage was another dismal possibility.

Treatment: Rubbing alcohol isode in *30K* potency, one drop. The boy was observed for 30 minutes and he appeared to be comfortable. The father was instructed to bring the boy to an emergency room immediately if the pain returned or the boy developed any signs of ill health.

Follow-up: The boy enjoyed complete recovery.

A case of pollution poisoning after the 1993 World Trade Center bombing

A young crew worker became very sick after inhaling noxious fumes at the World Trade Center following its bombing in 1993. He complained of difficulty breathing, sore throat, fatigue, and dermatitis. A pulmonary function test performed by his physician showed impairment of his lung capacity. A black sludge was removed from his throat by a specialist, who prescribed steroid inhaler medications. A dermatologist prescribed a topical steroid ointment. None of these treatments helped and he remained sick and disabled.

Bio-resonance testing indicated the presence of heavy environmental pollutants related to smoke inhalation, including carbon monoxide, in his respiratory and lymphatic systems.

Treatment: complex homeopathic remedy containing the same environmental pollutants, one drop, in 12X potency. The steroid inhalers and ointment were discontinued.

Follow-up visit: Two weeks later, he enjoyed 75% improvement in all symptoms.

Bio-resonance testing indicated the continued presence of mild residues of environmental pollutants, including asbestos.

Treatment: The same homeopathic environmental pollutants remedy was repeated, followed by treatment with the homeopathic *Asbestos 12X.*

Follow-up visit: Further improvement was noted, with few remaining complaints. The pulmonary function test was repeated by his doctor and showed improvement as well.

Follow-up Bio-resonance testing continued to reflect the presence of mild residues of asbestos and also lead.

Treatment: Plumbum metallicum 6X (homeopathic lead) and a repeat of the *Asbestos* 12X.

Follow-up: He recovered shortly after the final treatment.

Comment: This case also demonstrates multi-layer toxicity which can sometimes be encountered in cases of severe environmental poisoning.

A case of sarcoidosis

Sarcoidosis is a dreadful disease that destroys the lungs and other organs through an invasion of granuloid scar-like tissue. Its true cause is unknown in conventional medicine.

A young man in his thirties became afflicted with a very severe and progressive form of this disease, despite of a very high dose of oral prednisone prescribed by his pulmonologist.

Bio-resonance testing revealed a heavy fungal lung infection. The patient was an owner of a bakery and had been exposed to heavy flour dust on a daily basis for several years. Wheat flour is well-known for its fungal content.

Treatment: He was advised to leave an open one-ounce bottle filled with water out for several hours in his bakery. Considering the severity and chronicity of his condition, as well as his continuous daily exposure to fungi, the isode was prepared in high potency—500K—to be taken daily at the end of each workday.

Follow-up: He lives in Europe and has reported making such good clinical progress on this regimen that his prednisone dosage has been reduced significantly.

A case of a urinary tract infection

A young woman in her twenties developed symptoms of a urinary tract infection.

Bio-resonance testing: Silver amalgam was found present in her kidneys and bladder along with secondary bacterial *E. Coli* infection.

Urine culture: Confirmed heavy growth of E. Coli infection exceeding 100,000/ml that was sensitive to several antibiotics.

Treatment: Silver amalgam and E. Coli isodes with proper homeopathic organ support.

Follow-up: All symptoms disappeared. Urine culture was repeated and read *"less than 10,000 nonspecific bacteria/ml. May represent normal flora contamination."*

A case of a "comatose" man

An elderly man in his 80's was brought in by his wife with a complaint that he had become virtually comatose over the last several months. He had not left his bed for weeks, sleeping through the day and night, and barely accepting food. He was unable to give any reasons for this. He appeared somnolent, vacant and very weak. On the surface, it was not clear whether weakness was the culprit or the result of prolonged inactivity. His doctor ran some blood tests and concluded that "there was nothing wrong."

Bio-resonance testing found lead contamination in the brain, adrenal glands and bone marrow.

Treatment: lead isode with appropriate sarcodal support.

Follow-up: Several treatments were necessary, as the patient was uncooperative about taking drops. Yet he recovered physically and mentally.

A case of medication overdose

A 78-year-old woman with heart disease took an overdose by mistake of a long-acting beta-blocker drug. The main pharmacological action of this drug is to slow down the heart rate and decrease blood pressure. As a result, she started displaying symptoms of acute hypotension which can be life-threatening in the elderly. She felt dizzy, clammy and weak. When she was examined, her blood pressure and heart rate were confirmed to be low.

The beta-blocker isode was prepared in several homeopathic potencies.

Bio-resonance testing identified 6K potency to be the most effective.

Treatment: Shortly after she began treatment, her blood pressure and heart rate increased and remained stable during several hours of observation in the office. She did not have to be admitted to the hospital and was able to go home.

Comment: According to official statistics, 750,000 deaths occur each year in the U.S. as a result of medication errors. Most of these involve the administration of the wrong medications or an overdose. In either case, the consequences of these errors could be greatly negated with the use of homeopathic isodes.

A case of double infection

A debilitated elderly woman in her late 70's was treated for a musculoskeletal problem and released from the hospital. Once home, she immediately began complaining of a respiratory infection, extreme fatigue and severe burning in her bladder, noting that she had had a urinary catheter placed in her bladder during the hospital stay. In addition, she had received a high dose of prednisone therapy, which is known to undermine resistance to infections.

Bio-resonance testing identified two infections: flu virus in the respiratory system and *E. Coli* in her bladder.

Treatment: E. Coli 200X followed one minute later by *Influenza 30X* and, soon after, *"Lymph-S."* A number of organ preparations for support of the immune and endocrine systems also were given.

Follow-up: Recovery was complete within 24 hours.

A case of respiratory anthrax?

During an outbreak of anthrax in the early winter of 2002, a middle-aged woman developed a high fever (over 102°F), chills, fatigue, and difficulty breathing.

Bio-resonance testing identified an anthrax infection in the bronchi.

Treatment: Considering the severity of symptoms and her good overall vitality prior to the infection, homeopathic anthrax—*Anthracinum*—was prescribed in a very high potency, 50M. Testing determined that this therapy would be both effective and well tolerated by the patient. She was advised to go to a nearby hospital in order to confirm the diagnosis, but she refused to subject herself to conventional medicine.

Follow-up, next morning: At least 20% improvement was evident.

Follow-up, 48-hours later: She was sufficiently improved to allow her return to work.

Recovery was complete within three-four days.

Treatment of nuclear radiation

In the late winter of 1996, I was awakened from a sound sleep at four o'clock in the morning—in severe distress caused by excruciating pain in my throat. This was accompanied by a sensation of sudden and imminent suffocation. My first thought was that it was just a nightmare, and that moments later I would be able to resume my sleep. But unfortunately, it wasn't a nightmare. The pain was real, and while I had suffered from my share of very painful throat infections in childhood, I never had experienced pain like this before. It felt as if burning coals had become lodged in my throat, leaving it with barely any opening to breathe. It also felt extremely dry, yet swallowing triggered excruciating pain. After realizing that this was a serious situation, my concern was how much time remained before I would run out of oxygen. My first impulse was to call an ambulance and ship myself to an emergency room. However, I still had sufficient oxygen left in me to realize that the condition was too weird and my allopathic colleagues would either pump me up with cortisone and antibiotics or intubate my throat. None of those options appealed to me. I ran, or rather crawled, toward my homeopathic emergency kit, which contained many remedies, hoping that God would lead me somehow to the right remedy, as I was literally incapable of thinking clearly. My mind was pleading for a remedy to address—"fire in the throat, fire in the throat . . ."—and as it happened, I reached into my kit and somehow pulled out *Belladona 30C* as if some guiding force had responded.

I remember throwing some pellets into my mouth and waiting a minute or two to see if the remedy was doing anything or if I would be forced to dial 911 after all. I recall that the original sense of danger along with that terrible pain began to ease up somewhat and then I found myself being awakened by the bright morning sun. It was only after I awakened fully that I realized that the "burning coals" were gone, leaving behind only a sensation of mild heat in my throat and also a general feeling of malaise. An hour later, I arrived at my Long Island office in Westbury and decided to check myself with Bio-resonance testing to determine the origin of this bizarre episode. I screened myself against numerous viruses and bacteria, then toxic chemicals and metals. None of these gave any indication of being the culprit. I then proceeded to test any other toxic elements contained in my homeopathic test kit. Finally, the test suggested nuclear radiation was the cause of my illness. I recalled a very recent long drive in which I had passed through several New England states, thinking that I might have been exposed to a possible leak from some nuclear power plant along the way. "Well," I decided, "once I have a minute, I will make a homeopathic autoisode out of my own urine and it will end the radiation affair." Yet as the day progressed, I decided to postpone turning my raw resources into remedies. We began getting an unusually high number of emergency calls. Everybody, it seemed, even some with very robust constitutions, were developing very sore throats with much heat, swollen lymph nodes and severe weakness. Bio-resonance testing confirmed that all of these cases represented radiation illness.

The source seemed to be local, somewhere on Long Island, with most of the affected patients coming from Eastern end. If my testing results were correct, then the air alone would be a sufficient source for the preparation of the proper homeopathic antidote. The great majority of the afflicted, myself included, needed the homeopathic antidote—*"Long Island Air Remedy"* in *12K* or *30K* potency. In order to confirm that atmospheric fallout was the cause, no other remedies that might potentially be therapeutic were used. Practically everyone responded to the "air remedy" alone. I considered this not to have been a placebo effect because I projected a non-committal attitude with statements such as, "it appears to be" or "it seems to be" that atmospheric fallout was causing their symptoms, while always conveying the possibility that the remedy might be ineffective. I encouraged the patients to return for reevaluation should their symptoms persist.

During the next year or so, the fallout occasionally recurred. There was an incredibly high epidemic of a "flu" that year, at least on Long Island, and a 15-year-old boy and another member of his family developed pneumonia in the middle of July, which was highly unusual. The family happened to reside near the suspected source of the fallout. A "bad flu" was the official medical diagnosis by conventional doctors who were unable to pinpoint the true culprit. The diagnosis of "flu" certainly was plausible because ionizing radiation is known to impair the immune system, which predisposes the body to secondary infections. However, following homeopathic treatment, the propensity toward infections declined promptly. The radiation isode also effectively cured the sudden exacerbations of chronic and degenerative diseases (diabetes, hypertension, angina pectoris, lung disease and others) that became rampant during that period as people's immune resistance declined.

Several months into the outbreak, I finally overcame my reluctance to contact the media. I had been certain that my methods of testing and my finding of radiation fallout would not be taken seriously. Unfortunately, I was right. A reporter from a major local newspaper was quite skeptical. Yet, some months later, the story of a ground leak of the fission products from the Brookhaven National Laboratory on Long Island broke in the media. Officially, the leak was very much localized around the laboratory and reached only local ground water supplies. The subject was very delicate due to the high population density on Long Island, as well as potential liability issues. Nonetheless, in the January 26, 1997 issue of *The New York Times*, lab officials admitted that "small amounts" of nuclear emissions had escaped into the air. Officials added, however, that the emissions were considered to be a "normal occurrence as a result of the routine operation of the lab's nuclear reactor."

Another case of nuclear radiation

A middle-aged woman became very ill after visiting her brother in another part of the state. She felt extremely weak and complained of a sore throat, low-grade fever, and enlarged lymph nodes in her neck. "This Epstein-Barr virus is acting up again, doctor" she said.

Bio-resonance testing: Radiation illness. When questioned, she confirmed that there was a nuclear power plant within a ten-mile radius from her brother's residence.

Treatment: "*Long Island Air Remedy*" 30K, followed by "*Lymph-S*" and homeopathic spleen support.

Follow-up: All symptoms disappeared within 48 hours. This scenario repeated itself on several occasions following her visits to the same area. Each time, the "air remedy" that she would bring along cleared the illness. As time went on, she stopped coming down with radiation illness following the visits.

Treatment With Your Own Body Fluids— Homeopathic Autoisopathy for Biological and Toxic Assaults

In the 17th century, a physician working on the medicinal use of bodily toxins wrote that *where there is the disease, there also is the proper remedy.*[308] Today, very few realize that modern vaccination practices that have successfully eradicated and reduced infectious epidemics are based on the homeopathic principle—*let same be treated with same*. This principle has been in medical use worldwide for several thousand years. In various cultures, treatment or prevention of chronic and acute diseases has routinely included the administration of one's own urine, blood, menstrual excretions, bronchial mucus, pus, stool, snuff of smallpox skin blisters, saliva of a rabid dog or snake venoms. Several centuries before the discovery by Robert Koch of the bacterium causing tuberculosis, an Irish Jesuit, Robert Fludd, reported successful treatment of tuberculosis with diluted sputum of affected patients.[309] Likewise, successful accounts of using pus from smallpox blisters, dried contents of lesions of bubonic plague, blood of people infected with measles and other similar fluids in the treatment of infectious diseases can be found throughout medical history.[310,311]

It is also well-worth mentioning that conventional medicine is not adverse to using one's own ("autologous") diseased body tissue for medicinal purposes. For example, the newest hope for a cancer cure is the preparation of cancer vaccines from a patient's own cancerous cells.[312] It is of interest that conventional medicine also uses bodily fluids for medical purposes by extracting female hormones ("hormonal replacement therapy") from horse urine. In recent experiments in animals and humans, promising results have been achieved in the treatment of autoimmune diseases using antigens derived from body fluids.[313,314]

Homeopathy has elevated the principle of *let same be treated with same* to a higher and inarguably more aesthetic level, extracting only the energetic imprints of the actual bodily toxins. In addition, homeopathic remedies have been found to be far more effective in delivering an amplified and stronger stimulus to the organism in order to elicit a much better immune or detoxifying response.

Over the years, homeopathic remedies and vaccines have been prepared from the discharges or lesions of people or animals infected with anthrax, plague, syphilis, smallpox, gonorrhea, diphtheria, scarlatina, tuberculosis, pertussis, measles, rabies, and other infectious diseases. Virtually any attempt at toxicological and biological warfare, even with mutated, antibiotic-resistant, rare or highly lethal biological organisms can be countered.

Without a doubt, homeopathic autoisopathy, as well as isopathy, can be life-saving when other homeopathic or conventional treatments are not readily available. These remedies can be prepared utilizing Korsakov's method, as described in the previous section. Depending what physiological system is most affected, a corresponding discharge or body fluid can be used to prepare the remedy.

In cases of upper or lower respiratory ailments, sinus discharge or deep raised sputum can be employed. If urinary or gastrointestinal symptoms predominate, urine, stool, or vomit may be used. The amount of material collected is not that important—a quarter of a teaspoon will be sufficient for sinus and respiratory discharges and only a few drops of urine, stool, or vomit are needed.

When symptoms are more generalized and include fever, malaise, chills, weakness, body aches, lethargy, etc., it is the best to use blood. Alternatively, saliva or urine can be used, if you are not able to obtain blood through venipuncture. Even a finger prick may provide all that is needed, a drop, to prepare a remedy.

Sample collection

Blood

In cases in which a blood sample cannot be obtained from a vein by a qualified health professional, it can be obtained through a finger prick. Sterilize your skin first with an alcohol swab (available in local pharmacies). You may also purchase blood lancet stylets for finger pricking. If blood is to be obtained through venipuncture, a small tuberculin syringe with a tiny 25–27 gauge needle is sufficient. When collecting blood from a finger prick, it is better to prick a side surface of the tip of a finger. The harder the finger is squeezed prior to pricking, the less a finger prick will be felt.

Make sure the alcohol has evaporated and skin is dry prior to blood collection, otherwise the alcohol may neutralize a biological agent when blood appears on the skin surface and foil efforts to produce an effective remedy.

Squeeze a drop or two of the collected blood into a one or one-half ounce bottle filled ½ full of water and close the bottle tightly.

Saliva, deep sputum and urine

Purchase a standard plastic container for urine collection from a local pharmacy or medical-surgical supply store. You may collect urine, saliva or deep sputum directly into the container and then aspirate a few drops with a dropper and transfer them into a dropper bottle filled with water (as described before). If a deep sputum specimen is too viscous, you may use a cotton swab to collect the material, or the material should be wiped into a container and the entire content of the dropper bottle then added to the container. Shake the container vigorously for about twenty seconds. Then pour the liquefied contents back into the bottle, filling it no more than ¾ full.

Vomit and stool

Collect the specimen directly in the same kind of a container as above or in a large clean bowl and then transfer the sample into a remedy-making bottle using a dropper, a teaspoon, or a cotton swab.

Note:

Consult your local health department in advance concerning the precautions you must take in order to properly dispose of the residual blood samples, lancets, syringes, etc. Do not place objects contaminated with blood directly into the garbage.

If Bio-resonance testing is not available to determine the exact best potency for an individual, a minimum potency to use, prepared off excretory matter, would be 30K. Usually, higher potencies are preferable because in the case of autoisopathics we are dealing with impure agents in a more diluted form as part of a bodily discharge or fluid specimen. Higher potencies also will be safer because, in all likelihood, they will be void of a single molecule of the original excretions. With blood remedies, one has to exercise more caution as they act powerfully. 6K would be a starting potency for weak people, 12K for more robust constitutions, and 9K for the people in-between. Further management regarding waiting, repetition or resorting to a higher potency should follow the same clinical guidance described earlier for the use of homeopathic isodes.

It is necessary to add that in cases of higher potencies (30X, 30K and above, or in cases when digital potentizers are used, producing any potency magnetically), an autoisode prepared from one person can be used to treat other persons contaminated or infected with the same agent.

Before presenting summaries of a number of clinical cases, I wish to share with the reader that in my experience, homeopathic urine therapy was found to be the most effective in removing residues of nuclear radiation, whether the exposure was recent or had occurred in the past.

Clinical cases

A puzzling case

A 2-year-old boy had been ill for nine days. Always in good health previously, the boy deteriorated overnight and developed multiple severe symptoms: high fever with severe weakness, loss of appetite except for uncontrolled craving for sweets, intense bodily shaking, vomiting, deep wheezing and coughing. He also suffered from insomnia, incessant crying because of overwhelming fears, feeling hot with unquenchable thirst, and a bloated abdomen with profuse diarrhea. The father had taken the boy to an emergency room where the doctors could not establish a diagnosis and had prescribed cortisone with antibiotics in the hope that something would work. The father, however, refused to subject his son to drugs.

Bio-resonance testing revealed severe gastrointestinal infestation with worms and a viral flu infection. Upon questioning, the father shared that a few months prior to his son becoming ill, they had visitors from a Third World country who had brought some cooked "goodies" that the boy had eaten.

Treatment

- *Influenza 9X* (homeopathic flu virus), one drop
- Six hours later, *Argentum nitricum 12C*, one pellet (a constitutional homeopathic matching most of his physical and emotional symptoms)
- Six hours later, *Stool 30K* homeopathic autoisode, for the intestinal worm infection

Follow-up, 10 days later: The boy made a significant progress. The fever, vomiting, diarrhea, insomnia, thirst and loss of appetite all receded within 24 hours of treatment and were completely gone within days. Weakness, bloating, cough, wheezes and irritability were greatly reduced. The fears persisted, along with strong cravings for sugar, and the stools were not 100% formed.

Follow-up Bio-resonance testing indicated a mild residual infection with worms.

Treatment

- *Argentum nitricum*, one pellet, in higher potency, *30C*, due to persistent fears and sugar cravings
- Repeat *Stool 30K*, one drop, two days later

Follow-up, two weeks later: Three days after the *Stool 30K* remedy was taken, the boy expelled a large number of worms in his stool. He became much calmer and enjoyed a substantial improvement in energy level. His sugar cravings were greatly reduced but still present. The stool was not yet normal and his skin remained pale.

Follow-up Bio-resonance testing now revealed presence of nuclear radiation that caused immune suppression and prevented his immune system from completely responding to the stool 30K autoisode remedy. As the result, some worms still were present in the colon. Also, testing detected the side effects of a childhood vaccination, MMR vaccine, affecting the pancreas and disrupting his insulin regulation of sugar metabolism. (Mumps virus, a component of MMR vaccine in attenuated form, is known to infect the pancreas.) This pancreatic disorder contributed to the sugar cravings and the vaccine was placing a heavy burden on an important organ of the immune system—the spleen. The father confirmed that three days before the boy had become sick, he had received several vaccinations from his pediatrician. The boy seemed to be coming down with the flu at the time but the pediatrician said it was okay to vaccinate and refused to postpone the immunization, despite the father's plea to wait.

Treatment:

- *"Long Island Air Remedy"*, *12K,* for nuclear radiation
- *homeopathic MMR* 9X to neutralize the side effects of the vaccine
- *homeopathic Pancreas 3X,* two hours after the *MMR 9X,* to support the weakened gland
- repeat *stool 30K*

Follow-up: a month later, the boy had recovered completely.

Comment: This case serves as a good example of the complex and multi-layered origin of a seemingly common acute illness, even in a 2-year old child. Undoubtedly, allopathic treatment, without addressing the true causes of his illness, would have led to a risk of developing a number of serious chronic diseases, especially diabetes and leukemia.

A case of West Nile Encephalitis?

A young teenager developed symptoms resembling West Nile Encephalitis. He resided in New Jersey, one of the three states known at the time to have had outbreaks of this potentially fatal infection. He was suffering from high fever, severe headache, stiff neck and nausea. All of these symptoms are consistent with a diagnosis of West Nile Encephalitis.

Recommendation: Prepare a homeopathic autoisode, in 12K potency, from his saliva. If no improvement occurred within a few hours of administration of the remedy, the boy should be taken to a nearby emergency room.

Follow-up: The boy began to recover shortly after treatment and recovered completely within 48 hours.

Comment: Whether it was a case of West Nile Encephalitis caused by the West Nile virus or the result of infection with a flu virus could not be determined with certainty, but in either case, the therapeutic method was curative.

A case of bladder infection

A middle-aged woman complained of the symptoms of acute cystitis: severe burning on urination, steady pulling sensation, and discomfort in the bladder area. She was instructed to prepare a urine autoisode in 30K potency and to administer one drop. She was cured promptly.

Two cases of exposure to nuclear radiation

A 16-year old girl, a student in one of the private boarding schools in Connecticut, had suddenly developed enlarged lymph nodes in her neck without any other signs of illness. Her mother feared lymphatic cancer—lymphoma—and was advised by the school nurse to take the girl to an oncologist for a possible biopsy.

Bio-resonance testing indicated that she had been exposed to nuclear radiation.

Treatment: A homeopathic autoisode was prepared from the patient's urine, in 12K potency, as suggested by the results of Bio-resonance testing, and one drop was administered.

Follow-up: All of the enlarged nodes disappeared promptly.

A month later, the girl's brother, a student at the same school, developed similar symptoms plus debilitating fatigue.

Bio-resonance testing indicated that he also had been exposed to nuclear radiation.

Treatment: The same therapy produced the same outcome.

Comment: Within a year after these cases, two nuclear power plants in the state of Connecticut were declared to be "unsafe" and were shut down.

A case of reversed thyroid tumor and nuclear radiation

A 65-year-old woman, a former resident of the city near Chernobyl at the time of the accident and a current resident of Germany, developed a thyroid tumor thirteen years after the disaster. Urgent surgery was recommended by her German endocrinologists. She also suffered from chronic anemia and fatigue.

Bio-resonance testing revealed the residues of nuclear radiation in several organs, including the thyroid gland and bone marrow.

Treatment: urine autoisode in fairly high potency, 200K, due to the long-term chronicity of the problem, one drop, followed by homeopathic immune support. Shortly after, she reported a complete recovery. Upon her return to Germany, her doctor, a professor of endocrinology, after examining her new blood tests, inquired as to whether she received any therapy elsewhere. She was afraid to tell the truth. Her surgery was canceled, nevertheless.

A case of severe fatigue and nuclear radiation

A director of a filming crew for one of the major TV networks felt very sick and fatigued after returning from an assignment to the near-Chernobyl area. There she was tested by a local medical center specializing in radiation illness and found to have a high level of nuclear radiation in her body. A medical doctor in charge prescribed a pharmaceutical product to alleviate a problem but after several weeks she felt no better.

Bio-resonance testing confirmed that she was suffering from radiation illness.

Treatment: Homeopathic urine autoisode in 30K potency, followed by *"Lymph-S"* as well as spleen and bone marrow homeopathic support cured all of her symptoms within a few days.

Nights of the Tiger

After attending one of my seminars, a young Japanese health practitioner asked me to help him with the only health problem that he had—nightmares. He felt very drained by them because of their tenacious and violent nature. They would leave him feeling unrefreshed for the rest of the day and with a chronic sense of oppression.

In his dreams, he was always engaged in fights. One night, he would be fighting a shark, and another, his martial arts master. The consistent dreams that troubled him the most involved his being a tiger. The tiger would be pursued by either a pack of lions that wanted to rip him apart or by a group of men with rifles who were hunting him. He would either be running through the jungle, away from the lions, or lying low in the bushes, making himself unnoticeable to the men. These dreams haunted him for as long as he could remember. Being otherwise well-composed and rather introverted, he had tried to exercise the martial arts mind-discipline and also had resorted to homeopathic treatment in order to free himself from this nightly calamity, but all without success. Extensive questioning uncovered no psychological problems or traumatic experiences in his past.

Nevertheless, I was certain that Bio-resonance testing would reveal some suppressed or unrecognized psychological trauma from his past. Disappointingly, the testing proved me wrong.

Bio-resonance testing confirmed that his emotional center was intact. The only positive finding following the screening of his entire body was that his bone marrow contained nuclear radiation at a very deep level of DNA. I learned that at least one of his parents could have been exposed to the fallout that resulted from the nuclear bombing in 1945. Yet, to conclude that his dreams were even remotely related to this violent act of war would have been highly speculative. I told him that such a relationship could not be ascertained on a purely empirical basis. Still, the finding needed to be addressed or he might be at high risk of developing leukemia or cancer.

Treatment: High potency, 1M, (due to the genetic involvement) of radiation isode along with homeopathic bone marrow and *"Lymph-S"* support.

Follow-up: About a half-year later he reported that within 24 hours of taking the treatment, his nightmares had left him and never returned. On the whole, he became a calmer and happier person with a new sense of freedom from some unknown force in his life. He also added that he felt changed so much that he was still in the process of adjusting to the "new" him.

Treatment of Biological Agents with Classical Homeopathy: Clinical cases

A case of peritonitis

An unfortunate young man in his twenties with chronic kidney failure and diabetes was receiving peritoneal dialysis daily for ten years. As a complication of the dialysis, he had been suffering from recurrent cases of life-threatening peritonitis, over a 9-month period. Chinese herbs and acupuncture treatments combined with many nutritional supplements intended to stimulate his immune system initially reduced the recurrence rate. Recently, he had become much more vulnerable to these infections and was suffering from his sixth episode in the last two months. Each time he had to be treated with antibiotics. Unfortunately, for 48 hours prior to his visit to my office, he developed the same set of symptoms indicative of the onset of peritonitis: fever, chills, lethargy, fatigue, and foul-smelling pus draining out of his peritoneal dialysis opening.

Bio-resonance testing identified the presence of many toxic agents which, undoubtedly, kept his immune system in a state of suppression, fostering the recurrent peritonitis and which had caused his diabetes and kidney failure in the first place. Testing also uncovered a staphylococcal infection.

This patient presented a dilemma: Compromised kidney function precludes the timely excretion of the many noxious substances, particularly metals, and the isodes to fight the infection directly would likely not work fast enough in the presence of his severely compromised immune system. Therefore, a classical homeopathic remedy based on the physical and mental-emotional features of his disease seemed to be the only option—to avoid the use of antibiotics (for fear of developing mutated and antibiotic-resistant strains of infectious organisms). There are many remedies that can be used in classical homeopathy for peritonitis *per se,* yet only the remedy that would match a person's total picture would be effective. The patient's mental and emotional status was characterized by two main features: anxiety about health and his attempt to control it—an obsession with meticulousness and cleanliness. His extensive, meticulously organized, nearly 300-page thick medical file contained every detail of his medical history for the preceding ten-year period, including every lab test, medication, vitamin, herb or diet. His wife reported that he demanded she frequently change his dialysis-site dressings for fear of germs. His fear of infection also was reflected in a drastic move that he made, jumping away from my stethoscope in a state of panic and with an expression of horror on his face, because I might not have sterilized it before touching his chest. "It must be full of germs and they kill people, doctor!" he exclaimed.

Assessment: This patient suffered from a combination of systemic septic infection with foul-smelling pus combined with a state of intense anxiety for his health, including fear of germs and perhaps fear of dying. He tried to control all of these factors through obsessive-compulsive cleanliness and meticulous order. This type of presentation is best treated with homeopathic *Arsenicum album.* Bio-resonance testing helped to determine that this remedy would be effective in a 30C potency. The patient was told to take two doses that day and call back the next morning to report his condition. He was instructed to begin antibiotics and go to the nearest hospital should his condition worsen.

Follow-up. The next morning he phoned in and reported that overall he felt about 30% better. A day after, he phoned in and reported that all of his peritonitis symptoms were gone and he did not have to take antibiotics. The total time period for complete abolition of his peritonitis was 48 hours.

A case of pneumonia?

A middle-aged woman with the clinical signs of full-blown pneumonia—fever, chills and incapacitating cough—was expectorating noxious yellow-green mucus. The cough kept her sleepless for several nights. Neither cold air, wind, sugar, or smoking seemed to affect her cough. Instead, intense guilt centered around her husband's dissatisfaction with their new house would worsen her cough every night, when he was coming home from work. She would then isolate herself in a darkened room, where she would sit and cry.

Bio-resonance testing revealed that the dominant problem, interestingly enough, was not in the lungs but in her emotional center. The negative field was draining her energy and undermining her resistance to disease. The most effective therapy was the homeopathic remedy *Natrum muriatricum* in *200C* potency which, besides matching her emotions well—guilt, crying silently alone and suppressing her unhappiness—also matched her respiratory symptoms.

Follow-up: Treatment produced prompt and complete cure of both the guilt and infection.

Clinical Examples of Combined Treatment with Classical Homeopathy and Isodes

A case of severe bronchitis or pneumonia?

A young woman called complaining of severe respiratory infection accompanied by high fever and cough with yellow-green mucus. She felt very fatigued and nauseous with difficulty breathing and tightness in her chest. Breathing difficulties had made her cough all night long, precluding sleep. Because that winter I was detecting through Bio-resonance testing many cases of respiratory infections caused by a bacteria from the tuberculosis family—*Mycoplasma pneumoniae*—and known to cause nasty bronchial and lung infections, the isode of this bacteria was mailed to her.

While she was waiting for the homeopathic *Mycoplasma pneumoniae 60X* to arrive the next day, it was suggested that she obtain *Ipecacuanha* in *30C* potency from a local health food store. (An excellent remedy for relief of bronchial spasm and respiratory infection, particularly when accompanied with nausea.) She was advised to take it three times that day and, when the *Mycoplasma* remedy arrived, to administer 1 drop of it, once.

Follow-up: After treatment with the *Ipecacuanha 30C*, her breathing improved and became normal and she felt better overall. Most of the other signs of the infection, however, continued. Within 48 hours after being treated with *Mycoplasma 60X*, her infection had nearly abated. She was advised to repeat the dose, which ended her ordeal completely.

A case of severe abscess

A middle-aged woman developed a large abscess on her back. The pain remained intense despite the antibiotic treatment prescribed by her physician and was preventing her from sleeping. The physician told her that surgery would be necessary and advised her not to delay it.

The abscess appeared to be hot, red, and hard, and was oozing a small amount of pus.

Bio-resonance testing revealed immune suppression due to mercury poisoning with secondary bacterial infection. This particular infectious isode I did not have in my possession.

Treatment:

* Discontinue antibiotics.
* *Mercury solubilus 3X* followed by *"Lymph-S" 3X* and *Kidney 6X*.
* The next day: *Hepar sulphuris 12C,* a homeopathic "abscess surgeon" remedy for hot abcesses.
* Two days later: *Silica 30C,* a good homeopathic "abscess finisher" after an abscess has cooled off. This was also her constitutional remedy (as indicated by the totality of her genetically inherited features).

Follow-up: The abscess healed rapidly, although a trace of barely noticeable skin infection remained. A dose of another homeopathic remedy completed the cure.

A case of bronchitis

A middle-aged woman complained of severe chest congestion with burning and a productive cough of yellow-green sputum containing some blood. She was also very thirsty for cool water.

Bio-resonance testing identified *Mycoplasma pneumoniae* in her bronchi.

Treatment: homeopathic remedy, *Phosphorus 100C,* 1 pellet—for bronchitis. Repeat if necessary. In case of incomplete recovery after the second dose of *Phosphorus 100C,* proceed with *Mycoplasma pneumoniae 90X.*

Follow-up: She improved after treatment with the *Phosphorus* and recovered after a few doses of the *Mycoplasma pneumoniae 90X.*

Interestingly, her husband and two children also had similar bronchitis. The husband objected to homeopathic treatment and insisted on "real medicine"—antibiotics—prescribed by an allopathic doctor. Only one child responded to the antibiotics, while the husband and other child remained ill.

A case of encephalitis

A 46-year-old man developed a high fever, 102°F, with a splitting headache, stiff and painful neck, and generalized severe body aches. In addition, he was very weak, intolerant of light, and aggravated by movement. He was restricted to bed rest. Even the slightest jarring of the bed stressed him intensely. During his physical examination, he appeared lethargic, talking slowly and wearing sunglasses to protect his eyes against light.

Bio-resonance testing determined that he was infected with *Influenza virus type B* in the brain as well as other organs and tissues. The diagnosis of potentially life-threatening encephalitis was made. No specific therapy is available in conventional medicine for this serious disease and permanent neurological impairments might follow.

Although he was infected with *Influenza B virus*, the classical homeopathic remedy that matched the overall totality of his problems was *Belladonna*. The question was: Should the therapy begin with the *Belladonna* or the *Influenza B* isode? Bio-resonance testing suggested the homeopathic *Influenza B 200X* be given first and the *Belladonna 200C* be given in several repeat doses the next day. He was advised to go to a nearby emergency room in case of a lack of progress.

Follow-up: The patient's temperature came down to normal within 24 hours and before the *Belladonna 200C* was taken. The rest of the symptoms persisted. After several doses of *Belladonna 200C*, about 80% improvement occurred. A few complaints lingered. The patient was advised to repeat treatment with *Influenza B 200X* once. By the fourth day, the patient was cured.

A case of pneumonia

A 72-year-old woman with high fever, chills and a cough producing yellow-green mucus felt such overwhelming fatigue and lack of motivation that all she desired was to lie down and not even move her finger. Physical examination revealed coarse rales in one of the lungs. A chest x-ray confirmed a diagnosis of pneumonia.

Bio-resonance testing identified the presence of pneumonia with pneumococcus bacteria.

Treatment:

- *Isode Streptococcus pneumoniae 200X*, one drop
- *Phosphoric acid 200C*—homeopathic remedy for severe generalized state of debility

- High dose vitamin C, administered via intravenous drip—25,000 mg, with additional trace elements, for immune support
- Herbal supplements for lymphatic drainage and immune support

Follow-up: 48 hours after initiation of treatment, she had improved significantly. She returned home and saw her physician the next day, as she had been advised. Her physician recognized her improvement and did not think that it was necessary to initiate antibiotic therapy. Shortly thereafter the patient recovered completely. A follow-up chest x-ray confirmed the complete resolution of the pneumonia.

A case of a toxic strep

A young woman came in for an emergency visit with numerous complaints: high fever, shaking chills, pain in the throat extending into the ears, and intense pain, numbness and tingling in every bone and joint in her body. She was also experiencing difficulty breathing, enlarged and painful lymph nodes in the neck, pain in her kidneys, and extreme dizziness. Her feeling of fatigue was so extreme that she said she was not sure if she was even alive. She looked extremely ill and was unable to walk on her own from the waiting room to the examining room. She collapsed on the floor from exhaustion and needed to be practically carried into the examining room. Her family doctor diagnosed a severe infection with *Streptococcus type A*, the malignant type which causes strep throat, kidney, and heart complications. The infection had progressed to a very generalized and very toxic state.

Bio-resonance testing determined chronic poisoning with silver amalgam and mercury throughout her body and including the immune organs. This was causing severe immune suppression that predisposed her to infection.

Treatment:

- *Baptisia tinctoria 30C* remedy in repetitive doses for her overall general toxic state.
- *Silver amalgam 5X* along with *Mercurius solubilus 2X* and later on *Strep. A 120X*. All to be followed with proper excretory, immune and organ support.

A broad spectrum antibiotic was prescribed in case homeopathic treatment was not successful.

Follow-up: She recovered completely in three days. Antibiotic therapy was unnecessary.

Homeopathic Treatment of Environmental Pollution in the Aftermath of September 11

Asbestos poisoning

A Manhattan resident who lived several miles from the World Trade Center complained of tightness and pain in the chest.

Bio-resonance testing identified asbestos poisoning in the lungs.

Treatment: Asbestos 60X, followed by *Lungs 30X,* one drop of each.

Follow-up: Complaints dissipated within hours.

Another case of asbestos poisoning

A middle-aged man employed at the building right across from "Ground Zero" complained of difficulty breathing when climbing two flights of stairs and said he had felt weak and cold for more than a month. His symptoms had begun after September 11th.

Bio-resonance testing identified asbestos poisoning in the lungs.

Treatment: Asbestos 60X repeated every two weeks for as long as inhalation of smoke from the site continues.

Follow-up in three months: For several episodes, the patient repeated the *Asbestos 60X* as advised, and all of his complaints dissipated for a week or two, and then returned. After repeating the remedy on a periodical basis, his symptoms vanished. He was able to stop the remedy altogether, even while the smoke continued at the site, and has remained free of symptoms for a year since.

Mercury poisoning

A Manhattan resident felt ill one week after visiting the observation platform at "Ground Zero." He began experiencing fatigue, "brain fog", and burning in the chest.

Bio-resonance testing revealed mercury poisoning.

Possible source: Dust and smoke containing paint, plastics, and residue of fluorescent light bulbs.

Treatment: Mercury 12X followed by homeopathic organ support.

Response: All symptoms were abolished within 48 hours and did not return.

Chapter 10

A Brief Analysis of the Benefits and Limitations of the Main Homeopathic Approaches in Cases of Biological, Toxicological and Nuclear Warfare

It would be hard to overestimate the potential effectiveness of homeopathic approaches as remedies against agents of mass destruction. In a very informative book on the subject, *Living Terrors,* written by international expert on biological weapons, Dr. Michael Osterholm, and journalist of *The Washington Post,* John Schwartz, several likely and frightful scenarios are presented.[314a] Among them, tens of thousands of people who are sick or in panic are demanding treatment and overwhelm the existing medical and other public facilities converted for medical use; shortage of specialized life support equipment; inability to accommodate long lines of people waiting for antibiotics, vaccines or other medications; mob fights; anyone who has a sneeze assumes that he has been "hit" too, and joins the storming crowd.

With many, even if available, medical measures rapidly losing their effectiveness because of just relatively minor delays, these homeopathic measures that can be rapidly employed by people themselves will be potentially lifesaving.

Isodes

Benefits

- These remedies are highly specific in their ability to stimulate the body's defenses against any offending agent.
- They are exceptional for both treatment and prophylaxis.
- They offer excellent versatility because they can be prepared rapidly, even by laypersons, and work against unanticipated agents and genetically altered or mutated biological agents.

- Their versatility is particularly valuable under the circumstances in which an enemy is expected to use a biological agent, yet protective therapeutics are either scarce or nonexistent.

  For example, botulinum toxin, which kills its victims by inducing respiratory paralysis, poses the most serious threat to U.S. servicemen at the present time, according to Col. Eril Henchal at the Army's Medical Research Institute of Infectious Diseases at Fort Detrick, Md. He has said that U.S. Forces have no vaccine to counter the toxin. Furthermore, the supplies of an antitoxin that can mitigate the post-exposure illness "are scant."
- Isodes are best administered as early as possible in the course of a disease, before a more advanced state of pathology develops.
- For best results, isodes are to be followed by "drainage" organ support remedies, which enhance proper excretion of toxins released from the tissues, and enhanced hydration.

Drawbacks

- Isodes may not be as effective in more advanced stages of disease, particularly if disease is due to biological agents, i.e., very toxic end-stages of anthrax, smallpox, etc. This limitation may not apply to cases of illness caused by toxicological poisons or nuclear radiation.

Autoisodes

Benefits

- Autoisodes are the second most specific remedies to stimulate endogenous defenses against offending agents.
- These remedies are indispensable in cases of advanced pathological and toxic states, i.e., anthrax, smallpox, etc.
- Their versatility is excellent and comparable to that of isodes.
- Hypothetical concern regarding their potential to trigger autoimmune reactions does not appear to be justified; this has never been observed or reported, as the body discerns the energetic pattern of foreign invaders from its own elements.

Classical Homeopathy

Benefits

◆ This approach emphasizes individualized assessment and selection of a remedy that increases the individual body's defenses most appropriately.
◆ Classical homeopathy can be very useful at any stage and is particularly effective in advanced cases where most conventional medications have failed or are ineffective.

Drawbacks

◆ There is a shortage of skilled U.S. homeopaths in the U.S., due to the dearth of good homeopathic schools and training.
◆ In cases of exposure to highly toxic agents (i.e., sarin gas, nuclear radiation, heavy pollution, or combinations of many toxic agents), as was the case with WTC fallout dust, the need for more specific remedies (isodes or autoisodes) will be unavoidable.
◆ In my experience, in cases of toxicological poisoning, even though administration of classical homeopathic remedies usually enhances the excretion of these agents, the removal of such toxic agents from the body is usually not as complete as that following correctly prescribed isodes or autoisodes.

Genus Epidemicus

Benefits

◆ Well-selected remedies matching the pathology of the initial stage of an illness can be very useful in both initial treatment and prophylaxis.

Drawbacks

◆ It will be time-consuming to accumulate and analyze data initially in order to establish the general pattern of disease development and arrive at a consensus regarding the remedy of choice.
◆ The shortage of skilled homeopaths may further delay treatment.

Complex Homeopathics

Benefits

◆ Complex homeopathic remedies may contain several biological
   or toxicological isodes and be useful when the nature of the exact
   offending agent is uncertain.

Drawbacks

◆ These remedies are much less specific than other homeopathic
   remedies.

   All of these methods can be used to maximum advantage if they
are administered by properly trained health care practitioners who
possess a good working knowledge of the field; and more specifically, are used in conjunction with Bio-resonance testing.

   For example, let us consider homeopathic options against the
deadly chemical toxin, ricin, for which conventional medicine does
not have any specific antidote or treatment. Ricin is a poison that
can be made from the byproducts in the process of extracting castor
oil out from beans. This toxin paralyzes protein production by the
cells of organs, and leads to organ failure and death. It can be
weaponized as an aerosol, liquid to contaminate food, or can be
lethal even through a skin prick.

   According to the Center for Disease Control (CDC), it was al-
legedly used by Iraq in the war against Iran, and that CDC believes
it was possessed by Al Qaeda in Afganistan. Even a few micrograms
of ricin, which is many-fold smaller than the head of a pin, is sufficient to kill an adult. Depending upon the mode of exposure, a person dies rapidly between 36- and 48 hours. Only general non-specific medical measures are available through conventional
approaches while the person is dying.

   In an alternative scenario, a homeopathic isode can be prepared,
from ricin directly and administered swiftly as an antidote in cases
of exposure. If nothing else, one can prepare a homeopathic remedy
from several ground castor beans which would be expected to have
sufficient content of ricin. Under these circumstances, in order to
assure maximum chemical extraction, one ounce of 20–60% proof
alcohol can be applied for an hour or so followed by vigorous shak-

ing of the contents placed in a dropper bottle. From there, using Korsakov's method, described in the previous chapter, the remedy can be prepared. Should this not be made available, an autoisode can be prepared off ones' own body fluids, prioritized in the following order: blood, saliva, or urine, all of which would be expected to contain some ricin, regardless of the mode of contamination.

In cases of gastrointestinal exposure, vomit or stool could be used specifically; for respiratory contamination—deep mucus or bronchial aspirate. Classical homeopathic approach can be utilized as well, based on the patient's disease picture.

It's important to emphasize that no reliable conventional tests exist to diagnose ricin poisoning. This is very disconcerting for the sake of public safety as the necessary precautions or actions cannot be administered without major delays. However, with the help of Bio-resonance testing and a homeopathic ricin sample vial, the diagnosis of ricin intoxication can be established momentarily. With the assistance of FDA and CDC, a widespread response to community needs could be orchestrated.

Chapter 11

Anthrax and its Homeopathic and Conventional Management*

There are about a dozen and a half already or potentially weaponized biological agents that can be used against civilians or in military combat. They include bacteria, viruses, tick-borne agents, or various isolated microbial toxins.

In this and the next chapter, however, we will examine in greater detail only the two major and most likely agents for biological assaults—anthrax and smallpox. Homeopathic methods and experience presented in these chapters can be extrapolated and applied with certain modifications in the management of other biological entities.

Anthrax is an acute infectious disease caused by the spore-forming bacterium, *Bacillus anthracis.* Anthrax occurs most commonly in wild and domestic animals (cattle, sheep, goats, camels, antelopes, and other herbivores), but it can also occur in humans when they are exposed to infected animals or their tissue.

Anthrax is most common in agricultural regions, especially in South and Central America, southern and eastern Europe, Asia, Africa, the Caribbean, and the Middle East. When anthrax affects humans, it is usually caused by an occupational exposure to infected animals or their products. Workers who are exposed to dead animals and animal products from other countries where anthrax is more common may become infected with *Bacillus anthracis.* Anthrax in wild animals has occurred in the United States.

---

*Some of the data concerning anthrax was based on the information from the Center for Disease Control, Atlanta, GA and the Center for Civilian Bio-Defense Strategies, Baltimore, MD.

The disease may develop in three forms—cutaneous (skin), respiratory and gastrointestinal. The mode of disease transmission, intensity of exposure, and constitutional strength of an individual are the factors determining the form in which the disease will appear.

Cutaneous Anthrax

Cutaneous anthrax is the most common and most benign form of the infection. It usually occurs as the result of handling infected animals or their products (wool, hides, leather, or organs) and often in the presence of a cut or abrasion on the skin. It accounts for over 90% of all cases of human anthrax. Even though the symptoms can be very bothersome, the overall prognosis for survival is high, around 80%, even if left untreated. However, up to 20% of untreated cases may result in death. The signs of cutaneous anthrax begin with a lesion resembling an insect sting in the form of an itchy bump. Within a day or two, this may grow into a small blister, and then a painless ulcer, having a characteristic black, gangrenous spot in the center. The lesions also may appear as black or blue blisters, crusty oozing eruptions, gangrene, carbuncles, or boils. Often, lymphatic nodes or vessels may swell in the area surrounding the lesion.

Antibiotic Treatment of Cutaneous Anthrax

Conventional medical treatment consists of a prolonged course of a powerful broad spectrum antibiotic, Cipro, or one of a more narrow range antibiotics, Doxycycline. Either antibiotic also kills indiscriminately other, friendly bacteria in the body which are essential for proper functioning of our gastrointestinal and immune systems. This collateral damage, especially at the recommended length of prophylactic administration—60 days—makes many infectious disease specialists shrivel because the era of antibiotic resistant superbugs already has become an epidemic in itself. In addition, the astronomical cost—$72 for 10 days or $430 for a 60-day supply of Cipro—is a considerable factor as well. Furthermore, both the short- and long-term side effects, especially intestinal and systemic fungal infections, which conventional medicine often fails to recognize, are devastating. On November 9, 2001, in the midst of the anthrax scare, the Center for Disease Control and Prevention reported that in one study of 490 people treated with Cipro, 20% developed severe side effects, including the symptoms of life-threatening anaphylactic reaction, which manifested by skin itch and swelling of the face, neck and throat and led to breathing difficulty. Nausea and vomiting are other common side effects.

The serious diagnostic limitations of conventional medicine and the unwillingness of conventional physicians to accept responsibility for these iatrogenic (treatment-induced) diseases have produced this widespread epidemic of fungal infections which remain grossly neglected among conventional doctors. This is, according to *Medical Mycology,* a medical textbook on fungal diseases, despite "much evidence accumulated associating clinical disease with the use of antibacterial antibiotics."[315]

In addition, the recommended length of the 60-day antibiotic course is an empirical guess rather than a recommendation based on true knowledge. Dr. Miller of the National Institute of Allergy and Infectious Diseases acknowledges, *"No one really knows if a 60-day course of Cipro—what's routinely being prescribed as a precaution against anthrax infection—is necessary."*[316]

Considering these facts and the prolonged, but overall, not highly life-threatening nature of cutaneous anthrax, it certainly appears prudent to withhold antibiotic use and offer a trial of homeopathic treatment first.

Homeopathic Treatment of Cutaneous Anthrax

The first account of successful treatment of skin anthrax dates back to 1834, when Dr. Hahnemann treated a farm worker who handled livestock infected with anthrax and later developed a serious infection in both hands. Two drops of homeopathic isode *Anthracinum 30C* remedy cured him promptly.

Another farm worker was treated by Dr. Hahnemann for two anthrax pustules. Again, one drop of homeopathic *Anthracinum 30C* was swiftly curative.

The homeopathic remedy, *Arsenicum album,* has been observed to be very effective in homeopathic practice as the *genus epidemicus* of skin anthrax, particularly when the lesions turn black and gangrenous. In a book written by homeopathic physician G. H. G. Jahr, *"Forty Years of Practice,"* he described the cases of two farmers, each infected with skin anthrax that produced gangrenous lesions after cutting a cow. One farmer was treated with *Arsenicum album* and the other with *Anthracinum*. Both farmers were cured within 36 hours. In the 19th century Van Boenninghausen, MD, a world renowned German homeopath, used *Anthracinum* and *Arsenicum album* in *30C* or *200C* potencies for successful prophylaxis following exposure and treatment of anthrax. If *Anthracinum* or *Arsenicum album* is not available, an autoisode can be prepared from an aspirated or "popped" vesicular lesion. This remedy can be taken in 30X or 30K potency daily for three or four days. One can use the general rules for the collection of a specimen described in the smallpox chapter.

Inhalation Anthrax

The most feared manner of spreading anthrax is via an aerosol spray over a densely populated area and released from an aircraft as a biological weapon. The U.S. Office of Technology Assessment estimates that a release of only 100 kilograms, or slightly over 200 pounds, of anthrax organisms over Washington, D.C., might result in up to 3 million deaths. This would be similar to the killing power of a hydrogen bomb. In 1979, at a military biology lab in Sverdlovsk, in the former Soviet Union, 68 of 79 workers exposed accidentally to anthrax spores in aerosol form died. At the present time, we do not have a warning system to detect aerosol anthrax spores in the atmosphere.

Despite of the fact that inhalation anthrax is not contagious (it does not spread from person to person), its clinical course following a very long (up to 60-day) incubation period is extremely rapid and deadly. Initially the disease resembles a common cold, but death may occur within 24 to 72 hours. The greatest destruction is caused by several toxins excreted by the bacteria that rapidly destroy the lymphatic system as well as blood vessels in the lungs, resulting in blood clotting, extensive bleeding, and tissue degradation. Death takes place as the combined result of sepsis and lung tissue necrosis, complicated by hemorrhage and respiratory failure. Hemorrhagic meningitis may occur as well.

Gastrointestinal Anthrax

Gastrointestinal anthrax is considered to be the most rare and unusual form of this infection, particularly in the United States. Its course can be as ominous and as fatal as that of respiratory anthrax because it produces severe inflammation and destruction of the intestinal mucosa. Consuming undercooked meat of an infected animal is the source of disease transmission. The symptoms include nausea and vomiting with rapid progression towards bloody diarrhea, severe abdominal pains resembling "acute surgical abdomen," significant abdominal bloating with massive ascites (leakage of the fluid into abdomen), and sepsis. Death results from vascular collapse.

Diagnosis of Anthrax Infection

Conventional Medicine

• Rapid diagnostic tests exist but are not widely available.

Alternative Medicine

• Bio-resonance testing is capable of identifying the presence of anthrax infection in seconds.

Prophylaxis of Anthrax Infection

Conventional Medicine

• Administration of anthrax vaccine requires three injections under the skin, given in 2-week intervals, and then three additional injections after 6, 12 and 18 months. In addition, an annual booster is recommended.

Efficacy

• In experiments with monkeys, a high efficacy rate (88%) was reported against inhalation anthrax.

Complications

* Mild and local symptoms occur in 30% of patients receiving this vaccine, with slight inflammation and tenderness at the site of injection.
* Infrequently, severe and extensive swelling of the forearm may occur.
* Systemic adverse reactions occur in less than 0.2% of those receiving this vaccine.
* The vaccine has not been in extensive use and has been administered primarily to young healthy military personnel.

Availability

* Vaccine supplies in the U.S. are limited.
* There is no vaccine available for civilian use. Meanwhile, hundreds of U.S. military personnel have refused the vaccine for fear of side effects.[317]
* Not even the top biological weapon's experts of the U.S. Army know at the present time if the American anthrax vaccine will be effective against a genetically engineered Russian anthrax strain. It is feared that this strain can be replicated and used by any of a dozen nations and worldwide terror groups believed to possess this deadly weapon.

Homeopathy

Considering the disease's long incubation period, the administration of the *Anthracinum* remedy in *30C* or *60X* potencies, one pellet or one drop taken every three to four days, or in *200C* or *500X* potencies, one pellet or one drop taken once a week, should render adequate protection in the majority. Immuno-compromised individuals, such as those with AIDS, chemotherapy cancer patients, or those with chronic ailments of the immune system, should be assessed on an individual basis to determine the proper potency and frequency of administration. Evaluation by an experienced homeopath and Bio-resonance testing are invaluable in the immuno-compromised. I would recommend that they receive a much lower potency, 12X or 6C, every other day. This recommendation is appropriate for infants and young children up to 3 years of age. Older children, 3 to 10 years of age, may receive the *Anthracinum* remedy in *12C* or *30X* potency, one pellet or drop every three or four days. Children older than 12 should adhere to the regimen recommended for healthy adults.

In any segment of the population, the remedy must be administered less frequently should the remedy begin producing symptoms that are similar to the disease itself (this property of homeopathic remedies is called *proving*—the remedy has "proved" it matches the disease). For example, one of my patients who made periodic business trips to Manhattan during the anthrax scare was advised to take the *Anthracinum* remedy in *500X* potency at every visit to the city, but not to exceed one dose a week. However, he had to make more frequent trips at times and decided to repeat the remedy out of fear of catching the disease. Soon afterwards he began to experience low-grade fever, mild headache and cough. He was told not to repeat the remedy until all of his symptoms cleared completely and then to not exceed the recommended dose. His symptoms disappeared promptly and have not recurred.

The question might arise, "How would one determine whether symptoms are caused by the prophylactic remedy or by the actual disease?" First of all, in my observations, it is quite unusual for an actual infection to develop in a member of an average population who has been taking properly prescribed homeopathic isodes and has not been engaged in self-destructive behaviors. For example, for many years I have used a homeopathic prophylactic *flu vaccine* where I mixed together several main strains of various influenza viruses and bacterial agents, all in isode form, that are known to cause common colds and respiratory infections. They were mixed in 30X potency, to be taken twice a week throughout the flu season (from mid-fall until mid-spring). This homeopathic vaccine was given to everyone who did not wish to receive conventional flu or pneumonia vaccines for fear of the side effects of the vaccines. Recipients of the homeopathic flu vaccine included frail elderly people, and teachers who normally are exposed to many children with countless sniffles and colds. Very rarely did any of these patients develop respiratory infections during flu seasons. In contrast, on several occasions, flu infections and even pneumonia followed the administration of conventional flu or pneumococcal vaccines. One needs to remember that negative lifestyle factors such as excessive stress, substance abuse (alcohol, drugs, sugar, smoking), or lack of sleep, may impair both the immunity and vaccine action.

Regarding the differentiation of the symptoms of vaccine from disease, homeopathically-induced symptoms usually are mild and transient. True infection, particularly with anthrax, produces high temperature, sudden and progressive symptoms, and the deep sense that something is wrong. It is possible that symptoms of intermediate intensity could develop in someone who was taking *Anthracinum* or any other infectious isode or an *Epidemic similimum* remedy prophylactically when they became infected. Even so, this would result in the benefit of a more benign and limited course of disease, which anyone would consider to be a positive outcome. In my experience, the best and surest way to sort this out in seconds is through the use of Bio-resonance testing to determine whether real infection is present.

Treatment of Anthrax Infection

Considering the fulminant and malignant course of respiratory anthrax, both conventional and homeopathic treatments should be used.

Administering the homeopathic *Anthracinum* remedy would be considered beneficial only during the early onset of active infection—perhaps during the first 24 hours or so. Once the toxic stage has begun, with signs of excessive clotting and bleeding, respiratory problems, or meningitis and sepsis, neither *Anthracinum* alone nor antibiotics alone will be adequate. Undoubtedly, the palliative measures of conventional medicine aimed at the maintenance of vital functions would be very important in order to "buy time," while homeopathic therapy offers further hope for recovery. Homeopathy has two options to offer, even during the advanced stage of disease. One is the classical homeopathic approach based on the totality of a patient's symptoms, and the other is based on the administration of autoisodes.

It must be noted that classical homeopathy, as perhaps no other therapeutic system, has emphasized for over two hundred years the utmost importance of inclusion of the patient's mental-emotional characteristics along with the physical manifestations of disease. It is of interest that only fairly recently conventional medicine has also recognized the validity of the mind-body connection. This connection operates via receptors on the membranes of immune system cells which are sensitive to brain neurotransmitters. The immune cells themselves are capable of secreting neurotransmitters and hormones.[318] Another mechanism of connection lies with the energetic electro-magnetic brain wave-body interaction, whereby the harmonizing effect of the normal brain wave pattern has been found to have positive effects on body physiology. In contrast, brain-waves altered by stressful negative emotions, anxiety, depression, and fear exert desynchronizing energetic influences on physiological functions and health.[319] Prescribing practices that account for the totality of the patient, and that consider the mental and general characteristics of the sick along with physical disease features, make the use of homeopathic remedies very effective in the prevention and treatment of infectious diseases.

Here are some examples of the classical homeopathic remedies that can be used for the treatment of various forms and stages of anthrax, depending on the individual patient's characteristics:

Specific Homeopathic Remedies for Anthrax

- *Aconite*—high fever; dry, hot skin; thirst; restlessness and anxiety with a specific fear that death is approaching.
- *Apis mellifica*—stitching and burning pain with sensitivity to the least amount of touch; furuncles with much redness and sloughing of tissues.
- *Arsenicum album*—the skin is burning like fire with a purple-like spot that is turning black and gangrenous; swelling with a sensation as if boiling water were running beneath the skin; skin can also be cold, blue and very dry, peeling off in large scales; discharges are thin and acrid and from any orifice; cold sweat with frequent and weak irregular pulse; frustration with restlessness and anxiety might be present; a patient often is thirsty and drinks small amounts frequently; fear of death.
- *Belladonna*—phlegmonous inflammation affecting adjacent lymph nodes; meningitis with a hot-flushed face, stiff neck and delirium; delirium accompanied with violent movements.

- *Camphora*—skin tense, hot and dry like parchment; anxiety with great exhaustion and fear of being left alone; bad sores, threatening gangrene.
- *Carbolic acid*—gangrenous ulcers with sloughing of skin and terrible burning pains.
- *China officinalis*—profound exhaustion with excessive sensitiveness and irritability of all senses; especially sensitive to light, noise, touch, and being jarred; feeling of being cold; signs of tissue decomposition with periodic fevers and chills.
- *Crotalus horridus*—more advanced stages with bleeding or oozing of blood from multiple orifices; blood looks black, thick, tarlike and is decomposing rapidly with an offensive smell; high fever with very weak pulse and extreme weakness; jaundice; coffee ground-appearing offensive-smelling diarrhea; weepy, desperate; delirium; symptoms worse on right side.
- *Hepar sulphuris*—formation of boils, pustules and abscess around the anthrax lesion. This remedy has been known as the "homeopathic scalpel" for its ability to bring hot abscesses to maturity and rupture, relieving the pain through evacuation of pus.
- *Hyoscyamus*—meningitis and cerebral irritation; symptoms of anthrax accompanied by great restlessness and excessive nervous excitement; shaking of the head in all directions; closing of the pharynx; itching around the affected areas; visual hallucinations.
- *Ipecacuanha*—meningitis or other ailments when the symptoms of drowsiness and nausea are made worse by vomiting.
- *Kali iodatum*—severe distension of the tissue with underlying infiltration and much infection of the surrounding enlarged lymph nodes.
- *Kreosotum*—tendency to decomposition of the tissue with elements of pus and gangrene accompanied with debility that is improved by rest.
- *Lachesis mutus*—malignant cases of anthrax accompanied by black or blue blisters and dark redness around the sore; the lesions often discharge dark, bloody pus; extreme sensitivity of the skin with fear of being touched or approached by anyone, accompanied with irritability and restlessness; refusal to take medicine because of paranoid delusions with fear of being poisoned by a doctor or others; typically, symptoms become aggravated af-

ter nighttime sleep or even after a daytime nap; great propensity towards gangrenous development.

• *Lycopodium*—anthrax carbuncles aggravated by applications of warm compresses; sensation of burning stitches all around; alternating states of chilliness and heat; pneumonia often affecting the right lung.

• *Pyrogenium*—recurrent painful abscesses with much burning; sepsis accompanied by restlessness and lethargy; horribly offensive discharges due to tissue and blood decomposition; bruised and very sore feeling accompanied with frustration and restlessness; paradox in pulse: mild fever with very high pulse or very high fever with normal or only slightly elevated pulse. This remedy is considered to be a homeopathic antibiotic. It is prepared from spoiled meat containing a multitude of different bacteria.

• *Rhus toxicodendron*—carbuncles, accompanied with burning and itching around them; presence of vertigo with the sensation as if one were about to fall; stupor with pale face and pointed nose; convulsions; bloody or serous frothy diarrhea.

• *Secale*—painful boils filled with green pus, particularly when accompanied by symptoms of internal heat with external icy coldness and, despite very cold skin, a desire to be uncovered; weak but with ravenous appetite and thirst; bloody, thin and foul-smelling discharges, and uncontrolled diarrhea; violent muscle spasms with diverse sensations (numbness, tingling, burning, crawling); improved by uncovering and cool air and made worse by heat.

• *Stramonium*—pains so severe that a patient is trying to escape.

• *Tarentula cubensis*—anthrax affecting the back of the neck with burning and excruciating pain making the person sleepless; great frustration.

• *Tarentula hispanica*—dark red-purplish deep abscesses or boils; rapid progression with violent burning pains causing much restlessness; a choking sensation; very sensitive nerve endings; more complaints on the right side; a person displays uncoordinated movements resembling dancing as the result of intense restlessness caused by pain, and feels better by listening to music.

• *Veratrum album*—diarrhea with the sensation that the stool feels cold; abdominal colic; vomiting with intense coldness of the entire body; dehydration.

These remedies usually are used in 30C potencies, although 200C potencies may be required.

A more detailed discussion of these and other remedies would be too exhaustive for this book. There are a great many remedies that can be individualized. For example, for bleeding alone, homeopathy offers 225 remedies, 139 for pneumonia, 80 for sepsis, and nearly as many for meningitis. A skillful homeopath will narrow selection of these remedies, often using a computer model that factors in the details and character of each individual case. For example, hemorrhage with dark blood would require different remedies than that of bright blood. In addition, the absence or presence of blood clots, their size, the general state of a patient, and so on would further narrow possible choices until the best remedy becomes evident.

Here are two accounts that attest to the efficacy of homeopathy in bleeding, based on individualized prescription.

An 80-year-old lady who was taking the blood thinning drug, Coumadin, had her tooth extracted. Although she had stopped taking the drug several days prior to the procedure, she continued to hemorrhage from the extraction site for over 24 hours. Upon inquiry, her daughter indicated that the blood was bright red. The woman was also thirsty for cold drinks. I advised them to purchase Phosphorus in 30C potency from a local health food store and to have the woman take two pellets. After taking the pellets, the bleeding stopped immediately.

A young woman developed a heavy life-threatening hemorrhage in her uterus immediately following delivery. The bleeding was very profuse with dark, thick blood mixed with clots. Her blood pressure and other vital signs were deteriorating rapidly, while all of the gynecological measures administered to stop the bleeding failed. She was given Pulsatilla, one pellet, in a very high, 50M, potency. The very second it touched her mouth, the bleeding stopped instantly.[320]

Some of the best acting homeopathic remedies that closely match problems encountered in septic states are those made out of snake venoms.

Often, excessive blood clotting results in bleeding when many blood proteins, including those that assure our normal blood clotting, are being consumed in the process of generalized pathological clotting caused by the bacterial toxins. This ominous state is termed DIC—disseminated intravascular coagulation. Once the septic states reach the point of DIC, mortality rates become extremely high as excessive blood clotting causes necrosis and destruction of the numerous organs. It also results in profuse bleeding through multiple body orifices into internal organs.

Snake venoms are known to have a profound effect on vascular systems and blood clotting. This is why if some poisonous snake bites are not treated promptly, the mortality rate is high. Death ensues from severe tissue swelling, thrombosis with gangrene and bleeding all leading to vascular collapse. There are several homeopathic snake venom remedies for abnormal blood clotting: *Crotalus horridus* (rattle snake), *Elaps corralinus* (coral snake) and *Lachesis mutus* (bushmaster snake).

What follows, for example, is a case in which the use of homeopathic snake venom upheld the principle of the same cures the same and had a profound effect as a remedy on the vascular system, bleeding disorder and infection in a 54-year-old man:

A patient was bitten by a rattlesnake on his right hand. Shortly thereafter, he developed profuse bleeding from multiple orifices of his body: eyes, nose, ears, mouth, rectum and urethra. His pulse was very rapid and weak, respiration frequent—40 a minute, and the fever was as high as 105°F. As a result, his whole body was bathed in hot sweat as he slipped into delirium and unconsciousness. Conventional medical treatments failed to help. He was pronounced to be near death and beyond hope.

A homeopathic doctor brought in on the case prescribed Crotalus horridus in 30C potency dissolved in water, one teaspoonful to be given by mouth every hour. Twenty-four hours later the homeopathic physician found the man to be completely alert, without temperature, showing normal pattern of pulse and breathing, and without even a trace of bleeding. Furthermore, he was also displaying a healthy appetite and was asking for food. The remedy was continued just in case for another two days. The man recovered completely.[321]

It is of interest that drug companies are very much aware of the profound effect of snake venoms on blood coagulation and vascular

systems and are trying to come up with the line of expensive pharmaceutical products by isolating some active components of the
venoms and turning them into patented synthetic drugs.[322]

Autoisodes

The administration of autoisodes, prepared from a patient's own
blood and containing all of the bacterial toxins that propel the main
destruction of anthrax, holds particular promise. I use this method
only in cases of severe infections when Bio-resonance testing indicates that both the blood and lymphatic system already contain a
heavy load of toxins. As a rule, the patients were very sick, but the
method invariably worked well. The use of autoisodes must be followed by the proper homeopathic lymph drainage—with the
"Lymph-S" remedy—in order to prevent toxic overload of the lymphatic system, which is a key component of the immune system. I
have custom-made this simple but very effective homeopathic formula for the lymphatic system. Other physicians trained in my
method have found this formula invaluable in aiding the lymphatic
function.

Suggested potencies for the blood autoisode:

* very weak state—3K or 6K, ½ hour later—"Lymph-S" 12X
* weak state—6K or 9K, 1 hour later—"Lymph-S" 9X
* moderately impaired vitality—12K or 15K, 1 hour later—
  "Lymph-S" 9X
* mildly impaired vitality—30K or 45K, 1 hour later—"Lymph-S"
  9X
* overall good or only slightly impaired vitality—60K, 1 hour
  later—"Lymph-S" 12X

Blood autoisodes constitute very strong remedies and potencies
above 60K should be utilized only by experienced practitioners.

A few general guidelines concerning an assessment of a person's energy-vitality state.

There are signs that are indicative of a very weak or low energy
reserve:

* **Appearance:** somnolent, lethargic, stuporous, with pale and
  clammy skin

Even in the presence of infection, a person is not able to generate high fever and in spite of his very sick state, his body temperature may barely reach 100°F.

- **Mental-Emotional state:** poorly responsive, no desires, avoids interaction, can not maintain a conversation, comprehension impaired.
- **Respiratory system:** breathing shallow, voice weak, hoarse and "cracks."
- **Vascular system:** the blood pressure tends to be low, top (systolic) below 90 mmHG ; needs heavy covering, feels cold.
- **Musculoskeletal system:** movements are sparse, muscle tonus is weak and unable to exert pressure or to squeeze someone's finger or hand.
- **Gastrointestinal system:** thirst and appetite are very poor or absent; bowel function decreased or absent.
- **Urogenital system:** urine—pale, cold.

On the other hand, a person can appear to be very sick and poorly responsive, yet be able to tolerate and even require higher potencies. There may be several indications that a patient has retained enough energy for the higher potency:

- agitated state
- hot, flushed skin
- strong muscle tonus
- high fever—102°F, or above
- speaks or shouts in a strong or loud voice
- harsh or violent body movements
- pushes away the blankets or caretakers
- emits strong bowel sounds
- releases concentrated, hot urine

There are, of course, variations of symptoms which fall in between these two sets of polar opposites.

In case of a **positive response** following the blood autoisode and *"Lymph-S"*, refrain from giving any more remedies. Observe.

In the event that there is no response, double the potency. The only exception to this is if the original potency was 60K. In that case, go to no higher than 90K.

If recovery is incomplete and further progress has ceased, repeat the same treatment that resulted in improvement.

Wait between 2–3 hours from the time the blood autoisode is administered to evaluate the effect of treatment. Whenever the potency of the blood autoisode was repeated or doubled, follow through with *"Lymph-S"* to assure timely excretion of the infectious waste products.

Chapter 12

Smallpox and its Homeopathic and Conventional Management

Smallpox is one of the most devastating infectious diseases known to Man, claiming a 30% fatality rate in the absence of immunization. The diagnosis of even a single case of smallpox is to be viewed as an international health emergency. Worldwide, smallpox was officially eradicated by 1977, thanks to the immunization program. Alleged to be the last, the limited stocks of smallpox that remained in the U.S. and Russia were to be destroyed by June 30, 2002. This, however, has yet to take place. Meanwhile, Iraq and other countries capable of bioterrorism are believed to own it as a bioweapon. According to the author Richard Preston, smallpox, among other potential biological agents, can be easily altered, thereby defeating the existing vaccine and turned into "the biological equivalent of an atomic bomb".[323]

Smallpox is caused by the *Variola* virus and is contracted primarily via the respiratory pathways, by inhaling droplets from an infected person or through inhalation of suspended particles. These particles may remain in the area for some time and can even be carried by indoor ventilation or airflow from area to area. The virus also can be contracted through contact with contaminated bedding or clothing if they were subjected to open smallpox lesions. The incubation period (the time from the beginning of exposure to the onset of symptoms) is between 7 and 17 days, with 12 to 14 days being the average.

The most contagious stage begins with the outbreak of the skin or mouth lesions.

If a person who has not been vaccinated within 25 years or so was in contact with an alleged source of the virus develops a fever of at least 101°F (38°C) for no apparent reasons within 17 days following the presumed contact, he or she is to be assumed to have smallpox.

The natural history of the disease consists of several stages. It usually begins with symptoms of high fever, between 102°F and 106°F, headaches, generalized muscle pains particularly affecting the back area, abdominal discomfort, occasional vomiting, and a transient, blotchy red rash. After several days these initial symptoms subside and the actual smallpox lesions begin to appear as painful mouth sores progressing to lesions on the face and forearms. The lesions look like flat spots, and are firm to the touch. They multiply and spread rapidly to the trunk and lower extremities. Three to four days after their first appearance, these flat spots turn into vesicles— bumps raised over the skin surface and filled with clear fluid. Shortly thereafter, the vesicles may fill with pus and the fluid turns cloudy, becoming pustular lesions or hemorrhagic if they fill with blood. This stage may be followed by recurrence of fever.

In the case of an unfavorable course of the illness, death may ensue within several days, even before the actual smallpox vesicles appear. Death occurs as a result of generalized sepsis due to a host of secondary bacterial infections that accompany smallpox, *Staphylococcus aureus,* pneumonia, and infection of the brain or bones. People who have been immunized with the smallpox vaccine may develop no symptoms or have a milder course of the disease. At the beginning stages, it is easy to confuse the disease with chickenpox. The initial rash is similar in both diseases. There are, however, a few differentiating features to keep in mind:

- Smallpox lesions are identical and evolve at the same pace, appearing on any part of the body. With chickenpox, a variety of lesions can be seen at the same time: scabs, vesicles and pustules, and they occur within the same immediate proximity.
- Chickenpox lesions are much more superficial and tend to inseminate the trunk very densely; the opposite holds true with smallpox.
- Chickenpox almost never affects palms and soles; smallpox does.
- Chickenpox usually renders lifelong immunity; a recurrence of this infection is unlikely.

Prophylaxis

Conventional vaccination

Routine vaccination of children in the U.S. was halted in 1972 after smallpox was believed to be virtually extinct worldwide. Blood tests suggest that the protective effect of the vaccine begins to decline significantly following a 5- to 10-year period after its administration, as evidenced by a drop in antibody production. The immune resistance for those vaccinated prior to 1972 is uncertain.

Currently, the Center for Disease Control and Prevention does not recommend smallpox vaccination for the public because of the potential for serious complications. These include potentially fatal encephalitis, vaccinia—the smallpox infection caused by the vaccine itself—and in a small percentage, death. There have been at least five main groups of persons identified who are considered to be at particular risk for side effects of immunization:

- people with eczema or other allergic skin conditions
- patients receiving immunosuppressant chemo- or radiation therapy or high doses of corticosteroids
- HIV infected individuals
- people with hereditary immune deficiency disorders
- pregnant women

It is my opinion that the side effect rates in the case of mass immunization, including fatalities, would far exceed those of the past. Clinical experience, observations and official statistics indicate that the level of health and vitality of the American population has significantly declined over the last few decades. Several major factors account for this: the increase in environmental pollution, an unphysiologic diet incompatible with human genetics, the cumulative effect of the deadly silver amalgams from generation to generation, as well as suppressive allopathic treatments that prevent the release of any internal toxicities. These treatments, in fact, "cement" external manifestations of these toxicities, whether skin conditions or discharges, deeper into the body. Not surprisingly, there are new epidemics of chronic fatigue, multiple chemical sensitivities, obesity, diabetes, and multiple sclerosis affecting even children these days.[324–335]

Vaccinia immune globulin (VIG) has been used to treat vaccine complications and to administer to those for whom the vaccine is otherwise contraindicated in conjunction with the vaccine. VIG, however, is difficult to produce and cumbersome to administer. Its supply is very limited, sufficient to treat only 600 people with serious side effects.[336] As is the case with anthrax vaccine, the U.S. Army officials are not certain if the vaccine will be effective against all of the 100 varieties of smallpox virus stored in Russian bioweaponry.[337]

Conventional Post-Exposure Measures

If no more than 4–5 days have elapsed since exposure to smallpox, an emergency vaccination is recommended. This recommendation also applies to those vaccinated prior to 1972. This approach was shown to reduce the infection rate somewhat and to significantly reduce mortality. An exception is persons with known contraindications. For these individuals, homeopathic vaccination would be a very viable option.

Homeopathic vaccination

Variolinum, a remedy composed of infected smallpox skin vesicles, is usually recommended in 200C or 500X potencies, to be taken weekly for the duration of an epidemic. Lower potencies of *Variolinum* or any other additional homeopathic remedies are not recommended, with the exception of remedies given to the immunocompromised and to children under 10 years of age. For those two groups, the approximate recommended dose would be 30C or 60X, 1 pellet, to be taken every 3rd day throughout the course of an epidemic. The potency is higher than that suggested for anthrax because of the highly contagious nature of smallpox virus.

There are two other alternative remedies in case *Variolinum* is not available: *Malandrinum* and *Vaccininum,* the latter of which is made from actual smallpox vaccine. These two remedies are also used to treat the ill-effects of the conventional smallpox vaccine. They should be used only in cases of severe complications, however. Mild or moderate symptoms are not to be treated, otherwise the efficacy of the vaccine may become attenuated. In cases of *Vaccinia,* the best results are obtained with 2 pellets of either *Malandrinum* or *Vaccininum,* dissolved in 4 ounces of water, and given as 1 teaspoon every 2 hours until the symptoms begin to improve. Bioresonance testing should be used to determine which remedy is best for an individual patient. Otherwise, *Vaccininum* would be the best choice.

For prophylaxis of smallpox in the absence of *Variolinum, Vaccininum* would be the preferred choice, given in 200C, 1 pellet every 4 days throughout the course of an epidemic. *Malandrinum* should be administered similarly, in the event *Vaccininum* is not available.

The same order of preference applies to the immuno-compromised and to children under 10 years of age: *Variolinum, Vaccininum, Malandrinum.* If *Variolinum* is not available, *Vaccininum* or *Malandrinum* is to be administered in *30C,* or *60X,* 1 pellet every other day. Should a person develop symptoms in response to either remedy, it is not to be re-administered until all of the symptoms subside.

Homeopathic Post-Exposure Measures

These are suggested homeopathic remedies, with potencies and frequency of administration, in case of exposure to the virus:

Variolinum 1M, 1 pellet. This is to be followed 6 hours later by the homeopathic *"Lymph-S"* remedy in *6X* potency, 1 drop, to enhance excretion of the virus via the lymphatic system.

The next day, *"Lymph-S"* in *3X,* 1 drop, is to be taken in the morning upon awakening. 3 hours later, repeat *Variolinum 1M,* followed in 6 hours by *"Lymph-S" 3X.* The third day, repeat the second day's regimen exactly. The fourth day, only *"Lymph-S" 3X,* 1 drop, should be taken in the morning.

The remedies are administered over 4 days:

* Day 1: *Variolinum 1M,* 1 pellet; 6 hrs. later, *"Lymph-S" 6X,* 1 drop
* Day 2: *"Lymph-S" 3X,* 1 drop; 3 hrs. later, *Variolinum 1M,* 1 pellet; 6 hrs. later, *"Lymph-S" 3X,* 1 drop

- Day 3: *"Lymph-S" 3X*, 1 drop; 3 hrs. later, *Variolinum 1M*, 1 pellet; 6 hrs. later, *"Lymph-S" 3X*, 1 drop
- Day 4: *"Lymph-S" 3X*, 1 drop

All household members or persons who come in contact with the exposed person should adhere to the same regimen unless they have been vaccinated with conventional smallpox vaccine. The immuno-compromised, debilitated, elderly, and children under ten years of age should follow the same program, but with the potency of *Variolinum* reduced to *30C* or *60X*.

NOTE: The same general public health policy guidelines aimed at containing an epidemic *must* be followed strictly by everyone involved. All exposed persons *must* be isolated immediately. Household members who provide custodial care *must* wear face masks and latex gloves upon entering the room of a person under isolation. All household members should be vaccinated immediately with a conventional smallpox vaccine unless more than 4–5 days lapsed from the time of exposure or they will be at high risk of reacting to the vaccine. Under these circumstances, homeopathic vaccination is advisable. It also is advisable to obtain appropriate instructions from your local department of health concerning protective gear and necessary guidelines for hygiene so that necessary items can be stocked in advance.

If a person quarantined breaks his isolation and is exposed to the smallpox virus again, the entire homeopathic regimen should be repeated. Likewise, other household members should repeat the post-exposure regimen.

Anyone who has received conventional smallpox vaccine within the last 25 years would not require homeopathic vaccination or homeopathic post-exposure measures.

Diagnosis

Conventional Diagnosis

Conventional diagnosis is established via electron-microscopy of the smallpox skin lesions. However, considerable time can be lost because the incubation period is generally between 12 to 14 days, and it can take several additional days from the onset of a rash to develop the appearance characteristic of smallpox.

A weaponized aerosol spray containing the *Variola* virus may directly infect only 50 to 100 persons. However, 10 to 20 or more times as many people within a dense and unimmunized population will become infected every day that diagnosis is delayed, and with devastating consequences.

Diagnosis with Bio-resonance testing

Diagnosis using Bio-resonance testing can identify the infected carriers within the first few hours following an exposure with a skilled practitioner able to determine the site of an exposure, if necessary, as well.

In these and other serious medical situations, the guiding role of Bio-resonance testing cannot be overestimated. In seconds this testing can pinpoint the critically affected organs which require immediate support and can also test any therapeutic items for efficacy or potential side-effects in an individual patient.

Treatment

Conventional Treatment

Conventional medicine has no specific treatment to offer once the disease has developed. Some experimental antiviral agents, such as *Cidofovir,* carry prohibitive side effects. In addition, they can be administered only intravenously, automatically creating a potential mismatch between demand and the delivery. Antibiotics aimed to contain secondary bacterial infections and general supportive therapy do not significantly affect the prognosis.

Infected individuals, along with their clothing and bedding, should be isolated immediately. Due to the potential for widespread airborne dissemination of the virus within a hospital environment and hospitals' inability to offer meaningful treatment, home quarantine is advised.

Homeopathic treatment

Homeopathy offers remedies based on the three stages of smallpox infection: initial, early and advanced.

Initial stage—before the appearance of skin lesions:

* *Variolinum 10M,* 1 pellet, followed 6 hours later by *"Lymph-S" 12X,* 1 drop. Wait 3 hours to begin using classical homeopathic remedies, if necessary, in accordance with the symptoms of the disease present at the time. *Variolinum 10M* may significantly alter the subsequent course of disease toward more benign form even if further symptoms continue to develop.

* *Antimonium tartaricum*—should be used while the patient has a dry, teasing cough and before a rash appears. This remedy is also very useful when the general and respiratory symptoms dominate and smallpox eruptions have not yet appeared on the skin. In such a case, a person may appear drowsy with a bluish-purplish face and may experience twitching, confusion, severe throbbing headache (particularly on the right side), irritability and dizziness. Very often patients requiring this remedy have serious difficulty breathing, with much rattling in the chest. Because this remedy promotes the appearance of skin eruptions, the general symptoms improve significantly as lesions appear.

* *Belladonna*—best used when symptoms are characterized by throbbing headache (usually relieved by holding the head or tying a band around it) and a dry, red, flushed or purplish face, with intense dryness in the throat.

* *Bryonia*—best used when symptoms are characterized by high fever, intense thirst with consumption of large quantities of water and unwillingness to move in bed because it aggravates all symptoms. In such a case, the smallpox rash is slow to appear.

* *Mercurius solublis*—most effective when characteristic features are swollen glands in the neck, particularly the parotid glands, profuse salivation and greenish stools containing mucus.

Early stage—when skin lesions appear:

* *Antimonium tartaricum*—should be administered as soon as the lesions have been formed; helps to moderate the course of the disease.

* *Apis mellifica*—effective when the lesions are accompanied with intense swelling, heat and itching. The patient may have a characteristic lack of thirst.

* *Cuprum aceticum*—effective when eruptions are uneven and of different sizes; there is respiratory difficulty of asthmatic type due to cramping spasms in the respiratory tract. Cramps are experi-

enced in other parts of the body, especially in the calf muscles; the pulse is frequent and the patient may be delirious.

Advanced stage:

+ *Crotalus horridus*—best for generalized septic states with bleeding of thick, dark blood.
+ *Hammamelis*—best for the hemorrhagic form of smallpox with oozing of dark fluid and bleeding from gums, nose, rectum and genital organs.
+ *Lachesis mutus*—most effective during the septic state of the disease with general frustration, extreme weakness, stupor and bleeding with thin blood containing dark particles. In this state, a patient usually cannot stand being touched due to extreme sensitivity of the skin and nervous system.
+ *Hepar sulphuris*—expedites the rupture and drainage of suppurating lesions, abscesses and lymph nodes.
+ *Muriatic acid*—useful in advanced stages of disease with collapse and loss of control of most functions due to sepsis and bleeding.
+ *Phosphorus*—a very good remedy for pneumonia when a person is thirsty for icy cold water and mucus secretions are tinged with blood. Such a person also may cough up large amounts of bright red blood or have bleeding from other orifices in the body.
+ *Secale*—another good remedy for septic states with bleeding that is thin, watery and dark with continuous oozing and fetid odor. Such a patient is often very lethargic yet restless with icy cold skin and a notable feature of refusing to be covered. This remedy also is useful in the treatment of gangrenous wounds.
+ *Rhus toxicodendron*—used when smallpox eruptions turn livid, begin to itch and are sensitive to cold air. Characteristic typhuslike diarrhea may be present with slimy, foul and profuse stools with a cadaverous odor and that may contain blood.

The suggested potency for all of the remedies is 30C or 60X in 1 pellet or drop. For the best results, 2 pellets or 2 drops of a remedy should be dissolved in ½ of an 8 oz. glass and 1 teaspoon of the dissolved remedy should be taken every 15–30 minutes until progress is achieved. After this, stop further dosing and re-evaluate the condition. If the same symptoms reoccur—resume the regimen. If there is continuous change for the better in terms of symptoms and general state—wait until symptoms settle into a steady picture before deciding if further remedies are necessary. In case of worsening of symptoms, a current remedy should be withheld, and a new remedy considered. On rare occasions, potencies of 200C or higher may be needed.

The administration of *Variolinum* in advanced, toxic stages of the illness is not recommended for fear of aggravating symptoms unless Bio-resonance testing indicates its safe use.

The use of autoisodes

If *Variolinum* is not available, a smallpox autoisode can be prepared from a patient's skin lesions at any stage of the disease by using Korsakov's preparation method.

Collection of the specimen for preparation of an autoisode

1. Clean a vesicular or pustular lesion with an alcohol swab and let it dry completely. Do not break the lesion.
2. "Pop" the lesion with a Medi Point Blood Lancet used for finger pricking and squeeze the skin until fluid appears.
3. Harvest some fluid on a cotton swab.
4. Dip the swab into an already prepared half-ounce or one-ounce dropper bottle ⅔ filled with good water. Stir the swab around vigorously several times inside the water, remove it and dispose it into a special container, according to your local health department instructions. If you use latex gloves, dispose of them the same way.
5. Close the bottle tightly with an eye dropper and begin the preparation process.
   NOTE: In cases in which another person is involved in the collection process, as might be the case in caring for a child or debilitated family member, he/she:
   a) must recently have been vaccinated with conventional smallpox vaccine.
   b) alternately, should undergo a 4-day homeopathic program with *Variolinum 1M* as described in the section on "Homeopathic Post Exposure Measures". Should *Variolinum* not be available, the prepared autoisode in *200K* potency might be used, even if from another person; 1 drop to be taken daily for

3 days, followed by *"Lymph-S"* as described in the 4-day program.

c) must wear a face mask and latex gloves.

Suggested potencies of homeopathic autoisodes for smallpox

The same general principle concerning the potencies and frequency of administration is to be applied here as in the case of anthrax infection: The weaker the person, the lower the potency. The more vitality the person possesses, the higher the potency should be. Homeopathic education should guide these individual determinations.

There are general guidelines for persons with good vitality:

Day 1: Skin lesion autoisode *200K,* 1 drop; 3 hours later, *"Lymph-S" 30X,* 1 drop.

Day 2:

a) fairly good improvement—no treatment, observe.

b) mild positive response only—either further lymphatic drainage or a repetition of the autoisode is necessary. To find out, administer *"Lymph-S" 3X,* 1 drop, and wait 2 to 3 hours. If the condition improves, observe further. If no improvement has occurred, repeat the entire Day-1 program.

In the unlikely event of no improvement, prepare an autoisode from blood using the same technique described for preparing an anthrax blood autoisode. Follow the same general guidelines for their administration. Adequate hydration, at least an 8 oz. glass of water hourly, is imperative unless an intravenous hydration is provided.

Caution:

Avoid massage, except for some gentle body clapping in cases of prolonged bed rest. Massage may lead to spread of infection within the body.

Overall, there are about 25 remedies that classical homeopathy has to offer for the treatment of the various stages of smallpox infection. As is the case with anthrax or any other illness, an experienced homeopath can quickly narrow the remedy selection to the most appropriate choice.[338–341]

Chapter 13

Other Supportive Measures and Considerations

General Environmental and Toxic Factors

It is important to take into account the pre-existing immune deficiencies that commonly occur in the majority of the population as consequences of the lifelong accumulation of environmental pollutants. The most toxic are metals (especially mercury, silver amalgams, and lead), whose intoxications are rampant in the U.S. The effective detoxification must be carried out with the skillful administration of homeopathic isodes accompanied with proper organ support and under the guidance of Bio-resonance testing. First, discontinue the dietary and lifestyle habits that drain your endocrine and immune reserve: sweets, sugar and its substitutes, refined carbohydrates, soda and alcoholic beverages, recreational drugs and cigarettes. Likewise, the use of stimulants like coffee or strong tea more than once in the morning is discouraged. Make sure you are getting enough rest and sleep.

Avoid environmental factors that are known to sap your energy, such as sources of man-made electromagnetic fields: fluorescent lighting, TV, computers, video games, electric blankets, waterbeds and electricity-operated surgical beds and armchairs. If the last two are necessary to use for health reasons, keep them unplugged most of the time. Minimize time spent on the telephone and use a speakerphone in order to minimize exposure to energy-draining EMF's. Move your bed at least 2 feet away from wall outlets. Make sure that only outlets that are distant from one's bed are being used overnight. Move the bed to a different bedroom reserved for sleeping if the bed is near a wall that has a TV or computer behind it in the next room. Likewise, excessive electromagnetic fields may affect your bedroom if it is located right above a television set in the room below or a kitchen which is known to contain many electromagnetic appliances, or a water main or circuit breaker box. Keep the TV and other unessential electrical appliances unplugged when they are not in use or place copper wires or pennies (older pennies contain more copper) under your bed throughout its length in 2 to 3 parallel rows, spaced 4 to 5 inches apart. Remember, man-made electro-magnetic fields drain your energy. Do not be surprised if by following these measures you will find your sleep and energy much improved.[342] The use of a simple electromagnetic field measuring device would be helpful.

Also, while you are on homeopathic treatment, stop using magnets of any kind! Their "healing" prowess has been grossly exaggerated and their general use is unsafe. If you use them just for a local chronic pain, refrain from their use temporarily, if you can. Depending on the severity, the pain may be contained with natural remedies or pain medications. Even better, see an experienced classical homeopath or acupuncturist.

After you have received a conventional or homeopathic vaccination, avoid professional dental cleaning or elective restorative dentistry if you have silver amalgam fillings. Otherwise, released mercury and silver amalgam will place a heavy burden on your immune system, making your response to vaccines unpredictable and possibly resulting in serious side effects.

Organ Support

It is important to underscore that during the toxic stage of anthrax or smallpox or in any severe and life-threatening condition, many organs, particularly those of the endocrine and immune systems, are subjected to extreme and continuous stress. In the majority of people, these organs are already weakened from the stress of living and from the chronic health ailments that many suffer. Proper organ support, starting with the prophylactic measures particularly following exposure and continuing throughout the acute stage of an infection, is crucial in order to allow the body to respond to treatment. Recent discoveries in immunology have established that our immune cells are capable of acting as mini-endocrine systems, secreting hormones that are necessary to empower the immune action.[343] Should the endocrine reserve become exhausted under the stress of infection, or any other stress for that matter, a decline in immunity will follow. Appropriate support can be provided by other alternative medical modalities and approaches if they are used and integrated skillfully. For example, as I have consistently observed in my practice, the administration of "glandulars" or preparations of organ extracts even in oral form may significantly enhance immune system responsiveness.

Conventional medicine claims that organ-glandular preparations are not utilized by the body and are excreted rapidly, making these preparations good only for making expensive urine. Fortunately, the scientific and clinical evidence speaks to the contrary. Almost a half-century ago, a study conducted at the universities of Vienna and Heidelberg examined the fate of these preparations within the body. Glandular preparations were labeled with special radioisotope markers and their absorption at organ-specific sites was documented with the aid of an imaging technique.[344]

Since then, many studies have demonstrated the clinical efficacy of organ-specific preparations in producing favorable changes in blood chemistry. Positive results have been reported by investigators at the Brigham and Women's Hospital in Boston and at the National Eye Institute.[345–349] In these studies, myelin, the protective sheath that covers nerves, was given orally to treat multiple sclerosis and collagen tissue was given orally for treatment of rheumatoid arthritis. Most recently, very encouraging results have been achieved in experiments on patients afflicted with Type I insulin-dependent diabetes following injections of pancreatic insulin-producing cells.[350] Numerous studies also have reported positive responses to the administration of a variety of preparations derived from the thymus gland in patients with a wide range of immune system dysfunctions, including cancer and AIDS.[351–363]

Chinese Medicine

Traditional Chinese Medicine offers a number of organ- and system-specific herbal formulas. Those specifically targeting the vascular system are known to regulate abnormal blood flow and may help to contain hemorrhagic complications of anthrax or other infections that are accompanied by bleeding.[364]

Herbs

Several herbs, such as *Astragalus membranaceus (Astragalis)* and *Echinacea angustifolia* have been shown to display immuno-enhancing properties and can certainly play a complementary role.[365,366] Even though some experts caution against the use of *Astragalus* in acute infections out of concern for its stimulatory tonic effect, with the use of Bio-resonance testing, the optimum dose to avoid complications can be ascertained easily.

Another class of herbs from the *Ginseng* family is known to elicit beneficial immune responses and also increase vitality and resistance to stress by enhancing the endocrine system and metabolism.[367–371]

It is important to remember that the quality, therapeutic activity and shelf-life of herbs and herbal preparations may vary widely. Their potency will depend on the manufacturer's methods of preparation and preservation.

Supplementation with Nutrients

In my own experience, vitamin deficiency is relatively uncommon in the U.S., even with the typical American diet, perhaps, due to the fact that many vitamins are added to foods. However, deficiencies of minerals and particularly trace elements are quite common. This impairs many vital enzyme functions including the ones of the immune system. Supplementation with minerals, trace elements and vitamins is definitely helpful during stress or times of diminished food intake such as occurs during a severe illness. Cheap synthetic formulas are not recommended. When supplementing the diet, do not follow the rule, "the more the better," or the effects may prove to be directly opposite to the ones sought.[372] Remember, there is a limit to which the body can assimilate even a good thing.

If possible, it is better to obtain vitamins, minerals, and trace elements in separate general formulations and in encapsulated or powdered form as the powdered contents of capsules can be mixed with any soft food or drink to make them much easier to swallow, particularly for elderly or debilitated people and children.

Other nutrients may be therapeutic. For example, supplementation with the amino acid *Lysine 750 mg,* three times a day, may reduce the frequency and severity of herpes virus outbreaks in infected individuals.[373] Hypothetically, Lysine 750mg, might also be helpful as a prophylaxis and therapy for smallpox, as this virus is one of the herpes family.

Diet

The amount of food consumed should be determined by one's appetite and the gravity of an existing condition. Heavy meals and overeating should be avoided. Digestion itself consumes a great deal of energy, which may partially explain the appetite suppression that often accompanies infectious diseases. If, however, a person desires meats, they should be provided. Simple carbohydrates should be eliminated and complex carbohydrates should not be consumed in excess. Maintaining protein intake is important because stressful conditions, such as infections, are accompanied with high protein losses.

In cases of poor appetite and low caloric consumption, good quality and well-balanced dissolved powdered or liquid protein formulas would be a good source of nutrients and energy. Vegetable juices should be encouraged and some fruit, too. Adequate salt and fluid intakes are imperative to support proper functioning of the vascular system.

Optional

Acupuncture and reflexology may be utilized so long as the classical homeopathic remedies have not been used; otherwise, a therapeutic conflict may occur. If only isodes or autoisodes have been used, acupuncture or reflexology would be welcomed.

Emotional Support and Prayer

The therapeutic value of such factors as a pleasant environment, emotional support and prayer should not be underestimated, no matter how grave a condition is.

Chapter 14

Post Traumatic Stress Syndrome and Psychological Problems Following September 11th

Along with the ravages of increased terrorist attacks, another insidious epidemic has emerged since September 11th—that of posttraumatic stress. According to *The Wall Street Journal* of October 21, 2001, sales of antidepressants and other drugs for anxiety and insomnia have skyrocketed. During the month following September 11th alone, medical doctors reported a 33% increase in prescriptions of "coping" drugs, many of these requested by persons who had never felt their need before. In addition to their expense, such polypharmacy fosters numerous toxic side effects and the risk of long-term dependency and addiction.

The U.S., neuropsychiatrist and researcher, Donald Mender, MD, in his excellent book, *A Look at Paradoxes, Physics, and the Human Brain,* addresses what he sees as the epidemic abuse of these chemical agents. He emphasized that these "materialistic balms for emotional pain not only fail to solve psychological problems, but also may rebound to multiply them."[374] He warns that "they can often enslave patients more completely than do their illnesses."

In stark and beneficial contrast, properly prescribed homeopathic remedies do not produce side effects, do not lead to addiction or dependency, are very inexpensive and, most importantly, are extremely effective in neutralizing the source of a person's psychological torment—the desynchronized cellular fields of the emotional center in the brain.

Clinical Cases

A case of a scared bladder

Jenny was brought into my office by her parents several months after the attack on the World Trade Center. Her parents reported that she had suffered from inability to urinate on her own due to a completely "locked" bladder following the shock she sustained on the morning of September 11th. Her elementary school was located only a few blocks away from the World Trade Center. Looking through the classroom window, Jenny and her classmates were stunned at the horror of a plane crashing into the second tower. As flames gushed out of both towers, the children were ordered to evacuate. They ran out of the school building watching the sky in terror. Jenny, along with many other children, feared another attack, and screamed all the way to the bus. Since that morning, she had become unable to urinate. She was suffering from intense pain caused by her over-distended bladder.

A urologist had subjected her to many tests and procedures but, in the end, could identify only a muscle spasm of the bladder sphincter. He prescribed a medication to ease the spasm and relax the sphincter. While on the medication Jenny continued to experience a burning sensation before and during urination that the urologist could not explain. In subsequent months, her parents had attempted to withdraw the drug several times, but the problem of urine retention returned immediately and the drug would have to be readministered.

Jenny had also begun to experience persistent psychological problems. In addition to constantly reliving the frightful events of that morning, she had nightmares of Mayor Giuliani issuing warnings of the ongoing bomb threats and of Osama bin Laden hiding behind her bedroom door, waiting to kill her. She also saw a ghost that was doing such a terrible thing to her that she was even afraid to describe it. On the whole, she grew more fearful, anxious and insecure.

Homeopathic therapeutics offer two remedies to individuals whose shock of fear causes paralysis of the bladder with inability to urinate, *Aconite* and *Opium*. Both are known for their remarkable ability to remove the imprints of fear that torment a person.

There are several distinct features differentiating these two remedies. Most people who benefit from the *Opium* appear as if they have been shocked into a state of general mental and emotional paralysis and numbness. They look as if they have been overdosed with opium or some other narcoleptic drug; they appear numb, dull, forgetful, slow.

In contrast, patients who will benefit from the *Aconite* after experiencing a life-threatening event tend to remain flooded with adrenaline on a continuous basis. They become permanently anxious, restless, fearful, and easily excitable. Any stressful event (exams, dental visit, flying, or even the telephone ringing) triggers an overshot of adrenaline and more anxiety, anguish, fear of dying, palpitations, insomnia, or waking up in the middle of the night with a fear of suffocation. These people live their lives in a constant state of fright and flight. It is no surprise that, physiologically, one of the bodily sphincters may become "locked" as if a person was in a constant state of running away from attackers. (During actual flight from a threat, many bodily functions except those that are necessary for immediate survival, shut off completely.)

The features of Jenny's condition suggested that she would respond best to the *Aconite* remedy.

Bio-resonance testing favored treatment with *Aconite,* in *12C* potency.

Treatment: Two pellets of the *Aconite, 12C,* were administered.

Follow-up: A week later, the mother attempted to discontinue the bladder relaxant drug but the problem of urinary retention returned promptly. A few weeks later, Jenny reported some definitely positive changes. The burning sensation during urination was gone and she felt more confident, much less fearful, and was able to recollect the entire event of that morning with far less anxiety. Her nightmares, however, were still present. The assessment was that the remedy had worked favorably but due to the depth and intensity of the problem, a single dose was not sufficient to cure her entirely.

Follow-up Bio-resonance testing indicated that *Aconite 12C* was the effective remedy. Two pellets were repeated.

Follow-up: A few weeks later, Jenny and her parents reported that 48 hours following the repetition of *Aconite 12C,* her urinary bladder medication was discontinued successfully. Her urination became completely normal without a trace of retention. All her fears related to September 11th were gone and she could no longer recollect any nightmares.

"What if they blow up the bridge?"

A middle-aged woman became afflicted with intense panic attacks and fears for several months following September 11. The fears reached a state of frenzy every time she watched government officials on television issue a new terrorist warning. These psychological problems, no longer confined to her mind, seemed to have spread throughout her body. She started suffering from a number of physical ailments, including chest pains, heart palpitations, insomnia, and fainting. She saw a cardiologist who administered several heart tests and concluded that she did not have heart disease. She saw her internist, who prescribed a tranquilizer that failed to address her fears. In addition, she underwent numerous sessions with three psychologists who could only reassure her that she was "relatively okay" compared with how most of their clients were doing. She decided to stop taking the tranquilizer and turned to homeopathy.

An interview elicited the following facts:

Most of her fears surrounded the issue of "what if . . . ?" "What if there is a food shortage?" She acted on this promptly and filled her basement with cases of canned food. "What if the stock market collapses?" She begged her husband to sell off all the stocks in their retirement account. "What if there is an emergency evacuation and she was stuck on the narrow escape routes out of Long Island, at risk of being crushed by other cars and people?" She began packing her belongings and begged the rest of her family to run away to join relatives on a desolate farm in the South. "What if I drive over the bridge and the terrorists decide to blow it up, cutting off the escape route? Then, I will be stuck on the bridge?!" This thought hit her while she was en route to my office and she barely made it across the bridge, having to restrain herself from jumping out the window of her car.

Physically, she felt hot and craved sweets.

Assessment: Anxious, impulsive individuals tormented by constant fears centered around "what if?," with a particular emphasis on situations where escape is impossible, and tending to be hot-blooded and craving sweets, match a state of mind produced by homeopathic silver nitrate—*Argentum nitricum.* Accordingly, one pellet of this remedy was given to her in *1M* potency.

Follow-up. The patient was seen 5 weeks later and reported that by the end of the second week after administration of the remedy, she found herself feeling normal. Her anxiety, panic attacks, fears and insomnia were gone. Even the depression with the sudden impulse for suicide that she had previously experienced (and neglected to mention during the interview) had left her. When asked how she would feel now if she had to leave Long Island in a rush, in case of a terrorist attack, she replied that this would no longer be a problem since she had found the solution.

"Even though I would still prefer moving out," she said, "if something happens, I am not the one who is going to be caught in all the traffic with a bottle of water and a pack of crackers in my hands. Let others do it, I'll stay home. I believe I lived long enough and if something happens where I'd have to die, so be it. I have peace about it now, this is my land, I was born here and I'm not running anywhere!"

"Will we survive?"

A middle-aged Manhattan resident who normally is a very confident and assertive woman had not been her usual self for several months following September 11. She felt overwhelmed with fears centered around further terrorist acts. This triggered a general state of anxiety and fear for her own safety and the safety of her only son. The financial security became an issue, too. She felt depressed and cried often, but only when alone, so that no one would know of her moments of weakness.

Physically, she complained of swollen breasts each month prior to the onset of menstruation and of completely losing her normally high sex drive.

Assessment: A combination of psychological themes concerning her own and her family's safety combined with financial insecurity, while concealing her weaknesses from others, lest she loses her position in society, calls for the remedy, *Calcarea carbonica.* *Calcarea carbonica* also happens to be an excellent remedy for women who experience cyclical breast-swelling on a monthly basis.

Treatment: One pellet of *Calcarea carbonica* was administered in *200C* potency.

Follow-up: All problems disappeared promptly.

Weepy for the dead

A normally very industrious businesswoman living in New York City had felt shattered for the entire month following the September 11th tragedy. Uncharacteristically, she felt a lack of any desire to do anything, including work that she previously enjoyed. She would sit and weep for hours while looking at the obituaries that appeared daily as more and more bodies were excavated. She felt helpless and immobilized, crying all day while she ruminated unsuccessfully about how she might help other people.

Assessment: A combination of sympathy for others with a lack of any motivation or activity, following an onset of acute grief or shock, calls for the remedy, *Phosphoric acid.*

Bio-resonance testing indicated that even a low potency *6C*, of *Phosphoric acid* would be effective under the circumstances.

Follow-up: Five weeks later, she reported that shortly after taking the remedy she was back to being her usual self. She had returned to work and had resumed her life as usual.

"What will happen to me?"

A young female émigré from a Third World country was consumed with intense anxiety, fears and sleepless nights following September 11. She had originally come to America to obtain the safety and security that she had lacked in her own country, where she always feared for her life because of the high crime rate in the poor neighborhood where she lived. After arriving in the United States, she had found and enjoyed safety for years until the terrorists demolished this comforting perception of hers on that tragic day. She did not wish to share her feelings with anybody other than her husband and me and felt she needed to repress her fears at work. Physically, she complained of frequent throat infections and feeling chilly most of the time.

Assessment: Personal security issues, the need to hide weakness, frequent throat infections and being chilly match the statefield of the remedy, *Calcarea carbonica.*

Bio-resonance testing confirmed the appropriateness of this remedy.

Treatment: One pellet of *Calcarea carbonica* was administered in *30C* potency.

Follow-up: One month later she reported that all her fears of terrorists and the anxiety concerning her safety were completely gone.

Case of a broken heart

A young couple who were madly in love became engaged on Labor Day, just before September 11. She was a successful professional and he was a thriving businessman. Her office was on one of the top floors of one of the WTC towers and that tragic morning she was unable to escape. Her fiancé, Glenn, who happened to have an appointment at my office that very day, called to cancel it and sounded very alarmed. He said that he had just received a phone call from his beloved while her building was already in flames. She told him that some of her co-workers were taking to the stairways but she was going to wait for the rescue team to arrive and that she would be okay and would call him back soon once the emergency was over. It was over soon, but she never called. As a few more days went by and her name could not be found among the survivors on the police list or in any of the hospitals in the city, he realized that further search was futile and he would never see her again.

About a week later, when Glenn came to my office I could barely recognize him. Usually cheerful, confident and outgoing, always well-groomed and dressed, he looked completely besotted and crushed. He was dressed as if he had just escaped a fire himself, hurriedly grabbing whatever clothing and shoes he could put his hands on. He was wearing an unclean, badly wrinkled and mis-buttoned green shirt, an expensive blue dress jacket, contrasting red sweatpants, different color socks, and some old winter shoes. All of his wardrobe looked baggy, as if it belonged to a person who was at least two sizes larger than he was. Glenn had not stepped out of his house for the entire week, nor had he spoken to anyone or answered the phone. It was obvious that he had not eaten or shaven for the entire week either. He looked emaciated and appeared to have lost at least 20 pounds. While staring at the floor of my consultation room, with a glassy look in his semi-closed eyes, he said that he saw his fiancée coming to visit him every night in his sleep. She kept reassuring him and asking him not to worry about her because she was okay and at peace. "So am I . . . , I am in peace . . . , I am in peace about it, too . . ." But his voice sounded lifeless and peace appeared to be far from what he was really feeling. As I applied my stethoscope to listen to his heart, I had to withdraw it hastily. It was as if someone had suddenly grabbed it on the other end and begun pulling me down into an open grave. I never had heard a heart filled with the vibrations of so much pain and deep sorrow in every beat. On top of this, the beats were heavy, somber and long, resembling chimes of a church bell at someone's funeral. The only difference was that his heartbeats were not regular and it was obvious that his heart rhythm broke too, and he was having an arrhythmia.

"Are you sure you're okay, Mr. T.?", I asked. "I'm okay, I'm okay, doctor. She's okay, too. We are both in peace now . . ."

I was concerned that his statements about being in peace, considering his real emotional state, were ominous signs heralding a possible pending dissociation or severe breakdown. It was obvious that the deepest degree of sadness and grief that any man can ever experience from loss of a loved one was all entrapped in his heart as he was trying to numb his mind with a lullaby of "peace." In homeopathy, such a state calls for its deepest remedy of bereavement, which is made from pure gold—*Aurum metallicum*. It has been known for over 200 years in homeopathic practice that persons in a state of grief matching this remedy usually are doomed with an unfavorable prognosis unless they receive this medicine. *Aurum metallicum* is used for the deepest, darkest and most overwhelming states of depression in patients who, as a consequence, are often led to become alcoholics or commit suicide. Other captives become reclusive for the rest of their lives, lose any will to live, or become unable to derive any pleasure out of life. Their depression does not remain confined to their psyche but it also permeates deeply their entire body, destroying the internal organs, particularly the heart and the vascular system. As a result, they face high risk of heart attacks, arrhythmias, hypertension and strokes. Bio-resonance testing confirmed the need for this remedy and the choice of potency. The remedy was administered in high, 25M potency.

Follow-up. Three weeks later, Glenn was still grieving, but there was a definite change in his appearance. He looked groomed, and the numb, mask-like expression had left his face. His voice and entire presence were no longer remote. He appeared stronger and more "connected" and he had regained some weight. In conversation, he did not mention being "in peace," which was a positive sign, and admitted that he was grieving profoundly. Further exchange produced some other encouraging signs as he showed interest in other spheres of life by offering his analysis of the actions being undertaken by our government against international terrorism. He thought highly of the Bush Administration's handling of the situation and made positive remarks about the fact that those who perished that day did not die in vain and that their deaths would help humanity attain a better and safer world in the years to come. The rest of the conversation centered around God, politics, and world peace. All of these were indications that he was departing from the dangerous state of *Aurum metallicum,* was becoming more attuned to ongoing events and started moving back to his natural constitutional state (known in homeopathy as one of *Sulphur*). The hallmarks of the *Sulphur* state are creativity, talent for innovative ideas (at was evident from his business endeavors), tendency to search for an underlying meaning in life and propensity to theorize and offer their viewpoints on the broadest spectrum of subjects including politics.

Bio-resonance testing confirmed that *Aurum metallicum 25M* was still acting and his emotional center did not indicate that any further interventions were necessary at the time.

Follow-up two months later: More positive changes reflecting further progress were apparent. He looked more upbeat and was back to his usual routine, regaining interest in his company that he had completely abandoned, although he had come to realize that the company and financial success did not mean as much to him as it used to and it would not be easy to be involved in the business the way it used to be in the old days. He still had feelings of emptiness and he was unable to bring himself to consider looking for a new mate.

Bio-resonance testing indicated that *Aurum metallicum 25M* had run its course and that, energetically, his emotional center could use some further help as the *Aurum metallicum* state was not quite over yet. The remedy was repeated but in much lower potency, *1M.*

Follow-up: Six weeks later he had undertaken a major expansion and renovation of his company. He was able to retrieve all of the pictures of his perished loved one that he had kept hidden for months. Lately he had been thinking about taking some time off and traveling throughout Europe, but did not want to do it by himself. He would rather do this with a new mate, once he was fortunate enough to find the right person.

Follow-up six months and one year later: He continues to progress and cherishes his memories of his late fiancée.

Osama bin Laden does not live here anymore

A middle-aged woman was evaluated for chronic psychological problems originating in her childhood. She grew up in a household with psychopathic parents and was subjected to continuous violence, terror and mental torture for as long as she could remember. She was routinely abused and beaten, especially when she got sick, as her parents could not deal with sickness and would express their frustration by "letting her have it." In addition to being abused, she was not allowed to express her emotions. This led to multiple health problems, manifested as tremors, regurgitation of food, diarrhea and anxiety-depression which, regretfully, were only perpetuated by her beatings.

Sitting at the family dinner table was her biggest torture because she could neither escape nor hide. She would sit, so overwhelmed with fear of regurgitating her meal that she would do just that; vomit onto her plate. Because this would trigger immediate shouting and hitting, she learned to contain the vomit in her mouth while pretending that she was still eating.

Her mother tried to kill her once and her father threatened to kill her many times. One night, when she and her parents were having dinner, just a day before her 18th birthday, her father told her in a very calm voice, "Leslie, don't leave the table after you are done, because once I finish my dinner, we'll go outside and I will kill you." She knew he meant what he said. She wanted either to scream, or run and jump through a window but she could not even move her toe. She found herself paralyzed by terror. Her eyes became "glued" to his teeth and his plate, counting in horror the pieces of food remaining on the plate as every movement of his jaw was biting off whatever little time she had left to live. After the plate was emptied, her father took a long kitchen knife and ordered her out. It was a dark, cold and windy night. She wanted to go to her room to grab a jacket, but he said it was unnecessary because it would be over soon. Her mother did not say anything to her except that she had to wash the dishes. When she got outside, she finally was able to re-gain her instincts and screamed and ran. Luckily for her, one of the neighbors intervened and called the police. This saved her life.

Because that night could have been her last, she had never been certain since whether she was alive or dead. Having survived all the horrors of her childhood, she had to struggle afterwards to decide whether her life was true or surreal. She tried to discuss this with other people but "who was to say if they were alive, either?" Keep-ing appointments, particularly with doctors, was a nightmare. On those days, she would be overwhelmed with doubts as to whether she needed to bother getting ready to catch a bus or a train on time because "the whole thing" might be a play orchestrated by someone in another world, and the buses and trains were simply running un-derneath, between graves. These ruminations invariably would im-mobilize her until the last possible moment, when she would throw on some clothing in a hurry, hoping to still be a part of this world. When she learned that her father became even more deranged and killed himself, she felt guilty and somehow at fault.

During her later life, the specter of death continued to follow her as she narrowly escaped a number of violent events. In the 1970's, she happened to be in a foreign country that sustained a severe earthquake and was saved by a woman who pushed her to the ground and covered her with her own body, thereby protecting her from huge flying debris. She spent that night screaming hysterically until she lost her voice. On several other occasions, she had been as-saulted during a robbery, and rape and murder attempts.

The rest of her medical history included episodes of epilepsy, depression, anxiety, phobias, obsessive-compulsive disorder and in-somnia. She had consulted many psychiatrists and was taking nu-merous psychotropic drugs; however, the most they could do was reduce the number of seizures and help her sleep. Her mental-emo-tional state and overall quality of life remained extremely poor.

Treatment: As a remedy for the terror that she was still reliving and her uncertainty as to whether she was dead or alive, she was given the remedy *Stramonium* in a very high, *50M*, potency. She was forewarned not to expect an immediate cure but, rather, to expect a temporary aggravation of her condition. This would occur as her repressed fears, imprinted as painful pathological cellular memories were expelled.

Follow-up: Six weeks later she reported feeling very anxious during the two- to three-week period following the administration of the remedy. After that, her anxiety completely disappeared and her chronic fears, depression and obsessive-compulsive disorder began to dissipate. By this time, she felt that she had already made significant progress. She confided in me that some of her even more paranoid ideas (that she had not shared with me initially for fear of "sounding crazy") had vanished, too.

One of her paranoid fears concerned the new wave of terror that she had experienced since September 11. She was afraid to open her door to take the garbage out of her Manhattan apartment or go shopping, convinced that Osama bin Laden and his Al-Qaeda bandits were lying in wait in the basement of her apartment building for her. She feared they would follow her outside and kill her. She also was afraid to open the windows, or to breathe the outdoor air for fear of inhaling anthrax germs. For the same reasons, she covered her mouth routinely with a scarf on top of a breathing mask. She refused to eat in restaurants or buy exposed produce in a supermarket fearing possible contamination with biological warfare by terrorists.

Further follow up five months and one year later: She was happy to report that her fears and the overall catatonic state in which she had lived all of her life had finally lifted.

Comment: Well-prescribed remedies in homeopathy, particularly in very high *50M* potency, have been known to continue their healing action for as long as a year or more. She is expected to make further progress in regaining control over her life.

The saga of a fire captain*

Following September 11, a captain of the New York City Fire Department underwent a change of personality. Normally very

---

*This case was contributed through the courtesy of Nancy Gahles, DC, CCH, RSHom (NA), a homeopathic practitioner in NYC.

strong, optimistic, and with an extraordinary energy level, this still fairly young man, became irritable, depressed and fatigued.

"I have a sense of total despair of what went on—343 guys are dead and 50 of them I knew. We all lost them and their families. My spirit is wounded. Part of me died. This loss is devastating."

In addition to having to deal with his own bereavement and declining health, he also felt overwhelmed with the burden of suffering and loss that the families of his perished comrades had to endure.

"I know what the families are going through—the wives, brothers, sisters, children. I have a sense of despair. I can feel the pain. I keep thinking about them."

And then, on top of it, he felt guilty. "I wish I was doing more. There's so much to do. Visit the families . . . I feel responsible. I should be doing more, but I'm trying to hold down my end. I feel my stamina is down. I don't have the will to get up and go. I'm down, physically, tired. My energy level is down. I'm just tired, man."

"His moods alternate, doctor", his wife added. "At the funeral home, he called me his rock and at dinner he called me a bitch. At home, he'll just sit in front of the fireplace and stare into it for hours."

His state of depression and resignation was building and continued for six months until he realized that this was something he couldn't shake on his own. He turned to homeopathy.

Assessment: quoting books on homeopathic psychology, we have an injured state of mind with the following characteristics: *"ailments from grief; despair, despair for others; unusual responsibility with such horrible depression of spirits that there is an absolute loss of enjoyment in everything; feeling as if lost; weary of life; sadness, hopelessness."* [375] *"Serious, over-responsible and depressive individuals; their pathology expresses the tension between their sense of responsibility, their will and felt call to control people and circumstances, as over the existential limitations they encounter."* [376] *" . . . the individual placed in a position of honor or trust who, through some misfortune finds his reputation on the brink of ruin. In fact, it is due to the type, intrinsic, high-mindedness and delicate scruples of conscience that one encounters, at times, a dra-*

matic quality of his crisis of ego, as if a mighty oak were struck down with a single blow." [377]

If the remedy, *Aurum metallicum,* is administered to a healthy person, his mind will begin to experience a similar torment. *Aurum metallicum 200C,* 2 pellets, was prescribed to the captain on two occasions within a several month period. His initial response was, "What was that stuff you gave me? About a half-hour after I took it, I felt immediate relief. Relief, like a tranquilizer, relaxed. My whole body. This is pretty powerful stuff".

Further follow-up: "I have good energy. I haven't felt this good in years. The despair lifted. I can do things again. It was pretty amazing. I felt physically relaxed, like a Valium. Can I buy a bottle of that stuff?"

Several months later: "This is the best treatment I have ever received. I still can't understand how some two little pellets could have such a powerful effect on a person ?!"

Just very recently, the captain was promoted to the ranks of chief.

It was reported that there are more than 130,000 people in Manhattan alone who still suffer from Post Traumatic Stress Syndrome or depression following the September 11th attack on the World Trade Center.[378] According to the American Psychological Association, the true number probably is much higher.

Chapter 15

Homeopathy for War and Injuries

Whether as the sole therapeutic modality or, when necessary, in conjunction with conventional interventions, homeopathy is potentially indispensable in the treatment of the wide variety of physical injuries caused by military combat engagements, terrorist acts, criminal assaults and accidents. Homeopathic remedies would be recommended in many cases:

- burns—*Cantharis, Causticum, Phosphorus, Urtica urens ointment*
- burns of electrical power and lightning—*Phosphorus*
- burns from nuclear radiation—*Apis mellifica, Cantharis, Phosphorus, Radium bromatum, Urtica urens ointment, X-ray, nuclear radiation isode*
- bruises, contusions, concussions, injuries—*Arnica, Bellis perennis, Ledum, Natrum sulphuricum, Opium, Rhus toxicodendron, Ruta*
- injuries to the bones—*Arnica, Ruta, Symphytum*
- injuries to the nerves—*Hypericum*
- near-drowning—*Antimonium tartaricum, Carbo vegetablis, Lachesis*
- hemorrhage—*Ferrum phosphoricum, Phosphorus, Pulsatilla, Sulphuricum acidum, Lachesis, Elapsus, Crotalus*
- hemorrhage with shock—*Aconite, Arnica, Belladonna, Carbo vegetablis, Millilotus*
- wounds, gunshot, stabbing—*Arnica, Calendula, Ledum, Staphysagria*
- wounds, containing unexpelled foreign objects—*Silica*
- bone fractures—*Arnica, Calcarea phosphorica, Symphytum*

Urban Mathieu, MD, a board-certified emergency medicine specialist at Memorial Medical Center in New Orleans has asserted, after 20 years of experience in a modern emergency room, that "there's more healing in my 30C (homeopathic) kit than in the whole pharmacy at my hospital."[379]

It is fortunate but regretfully rare, however, to find a hospital administration such as Dr. Mathieu's which allows doctors to provide patients with the full benefits of homeopathy.

Clinical Cases

Case of unsuspected head trauma

An 18-month old girl with a severe genetic disease affecting her mental and neurological systems suffered from significant retardation and uncontrollable seizures. She was very lethargic, unresponsive to her mother and the family, and unable to establish eye contact with them. She exhibited grossly delayed development and experienced as many as five seizures an hour on a daily basis, despite the use of several antiepileptic medications. Her neurologists and pediatrician took the genetic disease to be the source of all of her problems and told her parents that nothing could be done except to increase her reliance on drugs.

Bio-resonance testing discovered unsuspected head trauma. The mother confirmed that the girl had fallen and hit her head prior to the onset of lethargy and worsening of the seizures. Her neurologist's examination, however, did not show anything abnormal. Several homeopathic remedies were considered to be potentially effective based upon the key features of head trauma, lethargy and seizures. One of those remedies, *Opium,* was determined by Bio-resonance testing to be effective in *12X* potency. One drop was given to her in the office.

Follow-up: Within days, she became alert and responsive to her surroundings. Her parents reported a significant reduction in seizures as well. During one year of homeopathic therapy she made tremendous progress in her mental, emotional, and physical health.

Her pediatric neurologist, who originally was reluctant to begin decreasing her seizure medications, has since reduced her dependency on drugs without hesitation and even encouraged the parents to continue with homeopathic treatment.

"Nice but stupid"

A teenage girl sustained a severe head injury in a car accident three years prior to a visit to my office. As a result, she suffered more than 70% loss of her cognitive abilities. She had been an "A-plus" student, but following the accident she became forgetful and unable to concentrate. She had difficulty retrieving the right words, comprehending, and following simple instructions. In essence, she became mentally retarded. In addition, she suffered from frequent headaches and chronic anxiety. "Our daughter is a very nice girl, doctor" said the parents, "She is very much liked in school. She used to be very bright. Since the accident, she's been acting as if she is stupid."

Conventional medical specialists could not help her. I observed her face lacked expression and she spoke in a low monotone. She was unable to give much of a history due to poor recall. Neither the parents nor the girl were familiar with homeopathy or could relate to it in any way.

Bio-resonance testing confirmed that her brain was still under the impact of trauma.

Treatment: Several remedies were considered and, because of her concomitant headache and anxiety problems, *Natrum sulphuricum* was thought to be the right choice. One pellet was given in 1M potency.

Follow-up: Dramatic change for the better was obvious within just a few weeks. Her face and entire demeanor came to life and she and her parents reported that she had become a different child—her memory, concentration and sharpness had returned by at least 80%. Her headaches and anxiety had disappeared. She became more confident.

Follow-up Bio-resonance testing indicated that *Natrum sulphuricum 1M* was still acting and suggested that its action would continue for a long time. In order to resist the temptation to prescribe the next remedy prematurely, a follow-up visit was scheduled for three months later. The family, however, in spite of my detailed explanations, was unhappy that this visit was "wasted" because I did not prescribe additional treatment. They never returned.

Significantly, this response is typical in cases in which awareness and understanding concerning homeopathy is poor.

A case of a blind man seeing again

A doctor was injured in a devastating car crash that killed his wife and children. He spent almost a year in a hospital being treated for multiple head and bone fractures. As a result of the brain injury and irreparable optic nerve damage, he remained blind for fifteen years following the accident, and with no chance for recovery, according to conventional medicine. He took some homeopathic remedies without effect. After being re-evaluated by more experienced homeopaths, the *Arnica 1M* remedy was administered. The man woke up that night, looked at the clock and saw the time— 3 AM. His vision has remained intact since.[380]

A case of reversed epilepsy

A teenage boy whose abnormal EEG confirmed a seizure disorder which had been present for several years, was being treated by the Chief of Pediatric Neurology in a major university teaching hospital. Despite medications, his seizures were out of control.

Bio-resonance testing discovered signs of head trauma, parasitosis and allergy to the additives and preservatives contained in his seizure medications.

Treatment: Arnica 1M for head trauma and herbs for parasitosis were administered. His medication dosage was reduced.

Follow-up: His seizures decreased in frequency.

Follow-up Bio-resonance testing found a brain free of trauma.

Plan: Taper off and discontinue seizure medication and repeat EEG.

Follow-up: Free of seizures while off medications. His EEG was normal with no signs of seizure activity. Many years later he remains free of seizures.

A case of an embedded foreign object

A teenage boy had the tip of a needle lodged in his buttock after receiving an injection in an emergency room. His parents refused surgical removal and brought the boy for homeopathic treatment.

Silica—a homeopathic expeller of foreign objects from the body—was prescribed in *30X* potency, to be taken in several doses.

Follow-up: There was no response.

Treatment: A much higher potency of *Silica, 200C,* was prescribed, to be taken several times.

Follow-up: The embedded tip of the needle came up through the skin surface and was removed.

A case of neck injury

A middle-aged man suffered a severe whiplash injury after his car was hit in the rear by a drunken driver of an SUV at a high speed. The pain and the neck impairment were so severe that the patient had to support his head with his hands any time he was to move his head. His cognitive function and overall physical state deteriorated, too. An MRI demonstrated disc involvement.

Physical therapy caused worsening of the symptoms. Chiropractic therapy offered only short-lasting relief. An orthopedist recommended considering surgery.

Homeopathic remedies—*Arnica 1M, Rhus Toxicodendron 200C,* and *Lachesis 30C,* taken in intervals, cured him completely.

Two bullets in the head

It was very uncharacteristic for Mr. C to be as late as he was for his visit. When my secretary called his residence to see if he was on his way, she was told by his wife that Mr. C was not coming to my office and was unlikely to do so again. Speaking through her tears, she shared the tragic story that her husband and his brother had been gunned down just a few days earlier in what the police deemed to be "a mob-like execution." His brother was killed instantly and Mr. C had just undergone surgery to remove two bullets from brain and neck. He was in a coma in the intensive care unit and his chances for survival were dismal.

About a year and a half later, as I was passing by our waiting room area in the office, I noticed a familiar face smiling at me. It was Mr. C. Instinctively I began extending my hand towards him for a handshake but swiftly pulled it back in anticipation that he might have been paralyzed and wouldn't be able to shake hands. I didn't want to make him feel uncomfortable. Yet before I was able to withdraw my hand, Mr. C grabbed it and shook it heartily.

Forty minutes later, I watched as Mr. C entered my consultation room. "Where is his walker?" I asked myself. "Why is he not using a cane? Why is his wife not supporting him—won't he fall?" I looked at him in wonder as he walked towards me. His movements were smooth and strong; his speech, vision, and facial expression were completely intact. I anticipated finding some signs of the handicaps expected as a result of gunshot wounds like his—blindness, deafness, paralysis, loss of speech, mental retardation, and so on. Maybe I had misunderstood something, maybe the gunshots went elsewhere, not in his head and neck, or the caliber of the ammunition was small? But he and his wife confirmed that the bullets had indeed lodged in his head and neck and the ammunition fired by the two executioners was hefty (9mm and 38mm), the kind normally used by law enforcement agencies. "I'll tell you this doctor," said Mr. C, "my neurosurgeon was just as surprised as you are now, but what can I tell you, it was just my luck, I guess, that I've made it in one piece."

"Have you had any residual health problems at all related to this?" I inquired.

"Well, my hearing in the right ear has not been good and on occasion, my vision gets kind of blurry and out of focus. And that is it. That's about all. I really can't complain much."

This story still puzzled me, particularly considering his age (70 at the time) and the fact that he had enjoyed far from perfect health prior to the attack. Amazed, I decided to go through his file and see what homeopathic remedies he had received during his most recent visit prior to the bloody event. His chart read that he had received two doses of *Arnica* in very high potencies, *10M* and *50M,* for a back injury. Luck was with him. He had administered the *50M* potency, known to act for many months, just two weeks before he was shot.

Comment: To many familiar with homeopathy, the "coincidence" of receiving a few doses of *Arnica* in very high potencies and subsequent exceptional healing proves the preventive power of homeopathy. Along with many other homeopaths, I have been dispensing Arnica in high potency routinely to my patients prior to any surgery, childbirth or major dental work. Invariably, these patients always healed quickly, experienced far less pain and avoided any complications related to bleeding and trauma. They often reported that the doctors involved in these procedures expressed complete surprise at these benefits. On one occasion, I received a telephone call from one of these surprised doctors—an orthopedic surgeon with the New York Yankees, asking me to disclose the identity of that "vitamin" I had given to one of our mutual patients before surgery. He had never seen anyone heal so rapidly. *"Arnica 1M"*, I replied. "Thank you," he said, "it was a really good vitamin, maybe I should start using it too." "I hope you will, doctor. Thank you for your interest."

It is to be noted that the probable relationship between the *Arnica* and Mr. C's amazing recovery is not meant in any way to detract from the efforts and high skill of his surgical team. Instead, it provides a glimpse of the full potential to be derived from the proper integration of both conventional and homeopathic medicine.

Chapter **16**

How Cost Effective is Digital Medicine?

In the realm of private practice, a solo homeopathic practitioner does not have the resources necessary to conduct a thorough cost effectiveness analysis. Such a cumbersome task would require the cooperation and assistance of the wide healthcare network, including the insurance sector.

Nonetheless, over the years I could not help noting the staggering disproportion between the enormous cost of health care in the U.S. and its overall dismal quality and output. The official statistics, a staggering $1.5 trillion spent annually for our medical care on one hand and the U.S. Senate Office of Technology Assessment conclusion that only 10% to 15% of all medical interventions and treatments are safe and effective speak for themselves. Such a disparity is inevitable when medical practice is based on amputated research models and diseases are treated with total inability to address their true root causes. This especially holds true in the care of the chronic diseases that have become epidemic in the U.S. today. In acute conditions, when the immediate, triggering causative factors—fracture, rupture, injuries and infection—are more obvious, the success rate is significantly better. Even so, with the skillful synthesis of alternative modalities (particularly homeopathy based on Bio-resonance testing) it would be far greater and the clinical course smoother and much less costly for individual patients and society as a whole.

Here is only one example from my practice where the patient himself volunteered to compare the charges for a short unsuccessful hospital stay with the costs of successful homeopathic treatment.

A 70-year old man with a severe blockage in his coronary arteries, along with a history of gastrointestinal pains and fatigue of 30 years duration was taking four medications prescribed for the heart and gastrointestinal problems. Over the last 2 months, the gastrointestinal pains increased in severity and were accompanied by cold sweats and nausea, resembling the symptoms of angina pectoris.

Bio-resonance testing discovered the presence of several heavy metals throughout the body, including the coronary arteries. In addition, a number of the parasitic and fungal infections were found in the gastrointestinal tract.

Treatment: Several corresponding isodes with proper homeopathic and oral organ support were prescribed for a total of a 10-day course.

Follow-up: After taking the remedies for only two days, the patient did not feel any better and admitted himself into a local teaching hospital. After a 10-day hospital stay with extensive diagnostic work-up and intensive treatment, no definite cause of his problem was found and he was discharged in essentially the same condition but with more medications to take.

Upon his return home, he decided that he had nothing to lose so he completed the homeopathic treatment. Afterwards, he improved so much that he could barely point to any residual symptoms.

Further follow-up confirmed that his gastrointestinal problems and fatigue completely resolved. One year later he continued to feel well and enjoy a good quality of life.

His 10-day hospital bill was $39,599.52. In comparison, his office bill for the first visit that addressed the evaluation and treatment of the same problem was only several hundred dollars. Unfortunately, this well-documented case is representative of the overall fiscal and quality patterns in modern American health care. One can only guess what his total medical bills added up to over the 30-year period of his illness.

There were a number of studies performed in Europe which demonstrated a clear advantage and cost-effectiveness of homeopathy over conventional medicine.[381]

The studies conducted in France, England, and Scotland confirmed significant economic benefits of homeopathy in terms of much lower costs of medical care, reduction in expensive prescription drugs, much fewer sick-leave days and, as importantly, superior clinical response and quality of life while under homeopathic care.[382–385]

One small study conducted in Germany on infertility in women yielded a staggering 30-fold cost superiority of homeopathic treatment over usually astronomically expensive conventional management.[386]

Another study, in the U.S., showed that homeopathy was also more cost-effective than other alternative modalities, naturopathy and acupuncture.[387,388] Yet the overwhelming majority of the HMO's and private insurers' in the U.S. continue to deny coverage for homeopathy while the insurance premiums covering far more expensive and often unnecessary or less effective conventional interventions rise at an astronomical pace.

Chapter 17

Homeopathy: Past and Present

Despite the increasing popularity of homeopathy throughout the rest of the world today and the popularity it enjoyed in this country in the past, most Americans still lack an understanding of this fascinating medical science and confuse it with other natural treatments.

Very few are aware of how many famous people in the U.S. and abroad have been ardent supporters and loyal patients of homeopathy: Great Britain's Royal Family, Goethe, Charles Dickens, Pope Pius X, Thomas Edison, Mark Twain, John D. Rockefeller, Sr., Mahatma Gandhi, Mother Teresa, Hollywood's Jack Nicholson, Suzanne Somers, among others.

A number of these people have issued very strong supportive statements:

Mark Twain: *"Homeopathy forced the old school doctor to learn something of a rational nature about his business. You may honestly feel grateful that homeopathy survived the attempts of the allopaths to destroy it."*

John D. Rockefeller, Sr.: *"Homeopathy is a progressive and aggressive step in medicine."*

Mahatma Gandhi: *"Homeopathy cures a greater number of cases than any other treatment."*

Mr. Rockefeller, who may, in part, have owed his long life of 99 years to homeopathy, called himself a homeopathist and donated generous grants for the advancement of the field.

Sir William Osler, MD, the man recognized as the father of modern medicine, acknowledged at a conventional medical meeting that *"our homeopathic brothers pursue very seriously the scientific study of disease."*

Many Americans will be very surprised to learn how popular homeopathy was in the U.S. at the turn of the 20th century. At that time, there were 22 homeopathic medical schools in America, more than 100 homeopathic hospitals, and more than 1,000 homeopathic pharmacies. Fifteen percent of all practicing physicians used homeopathy in their practices. Several prestigious universities, among them Boston University, the University of Michigan and the Hahnemann Medical College in Philadelphia included homeopathic education as part of their medical school curriculum. The very first National Medical Society in the U.S. was the American Institute of Homeopathy, established in 1844. The AMA was formed several years afterwards.[389]

The first women's medical college in the world, the Homeopathic Boston Female Medical College, was established in 1848. It took another 42 years, and a half million dollars in endowments to have the first female students accepted to the allopathic medical school of Johns Hopkins University. Professional homeopathic medical societies opened their doors to female colleagues decades earlier than did allopathic medical societies; The American Institute of Homeopathy welcomed women in 1871, almost 20 years before the American Medical Association (AMA).

Homeopathic physicians achieved another landmark victory in the field of social equality around that time. In 1861, President Lincoln's appointed Secretary of State, William Seward imported his personal physician, Tullio Verdi, MD to Washington. Dr. Verdi was a former Italian Revolutionary and a successful homeopath with a degree from Hahnemann Homeopathic College in Philadelphia. Thanks to his skills and personal charm, Dr. Verdi became a very popular physician in the capital and provided his services to many political figures.

In 1869, three African American physicians who had served in the Union Army were denied admission to the D.C. Medical Society because of race. With the support of other homeopathic physicians, Dr. Verdi successfully lobbied in support of legislation, which passed unanimously in both houses of Congress in April, 1870, and established the Washington Homeopathic Medical Society. The society admitted "any persons without exception on account of color."

In retaliation the same year, H. Van Aernam, MD, a leader in the D.C. Medical Society and a member of the AMA, who happened to be a federal commissioner of pensions, announced that only allopathic doctors would be entitled to receive federal wages as retained experts. This meant that all of the homeopathic physicians who were carrying out the same duty, would not be funded and lose their jobs. When Verdi wrote personally to President Grant protesting this, Dr. Van Aernam was fired.

Homeopathy was, however, not just making strides in the social life of America but had proved itself beyond doubt in the serious medical battles of daily life. Many homeopathic physicians produced far superior results in the treatment of acute and chronic ailments, literally driving many allopaths out of town. Also, homeopaths successfully treated the deadliest of infectious epidemics with high skill and excellence.

As a prominent AMA member said at a meeting in 1903, "We must admit that we never fought the homeopath on matters of principles; we fought him because he came into the community and got his business."

It was only logical that by the turn of the 20th century many educated people in the U.S. became both the consumers and enthusiastic supporters of homeopathy. Other well-known intellectuals joined the list: William James, Harriet Beecher Stowe, Daniel Webster, and Henry James, among others. James could not help expressing his positive feelings about homeopathy in his novel, *The Bostonians,* by having one of its characters assert that homeopathy was a true system. Many clerics expressed their support. Among them, Mary Baker Eddy, the founder of Christian Science, who proclaimed that "evidence of progress and of spiritualization greet us on every hand. Drug-systems are quitting their hold on matter and so letting in matter's higher stratum, mortal mind. Homeopathy, a step in advance of allopathy, is doing this."

Tragically, she proved to be wrong when she concluded that the "drug-systems are quitting." Drug companies and the medical establishment, protecting their mercantile interests, watched warily as homeopathy has advanced rapidly and decisively toward the forefront of the American health care system.

For medical doctors, homeopathy always has been a serious challenge, impossible to master without expending long years of effort. Most physicians have been unsuccessful in their attempts to master it quickly in order to meet the competition. It has been my longstanding opinion that it is much harder to become a good homeopath than it is to become a good conventional doctor. Many contemporary medical doctors and homeopaths agree.[390] In addition, after the long and exhaustive years of conventional medical training required to earn the revered title of MD, it is hard to contemplate that for the most part your training may have been misdirected.

William James, MD, a famous medical scholar and one of the founding fathers of American Psychology, spoke as a proponent of homeopathy in 1898, when he addressed the Massachusetts State Legislature to protest a bill which would have barred practitioners other than MD's from prescribing for psychological problems. James accused the medical profession of failing to consider therapeutic methods that originated from outside the orthodox ranks. Presenting the various therapeutic approaches, he stated:

> *"Some of these therapeutic methods arose inside of the regular profession, others outside of it. In all cases they have appealed to experience for their credentials. But experience in medicine seems to be an exceedingly difficult thing. Take homoeopathy, for instance, now nearly a century old. An enormous mass of experience, both of homoeopathic doctors and their patients, is invoked in favor of the efficacy of these remedies and doses. But the regular profession stands firm in its belief that such experience is worthless and that the whole history is one of quackery and delusion. In spite of the rival schools appealing to experience, their conflict is much more like that of two philosophers, or two theologies. Your experience, says one side to the other, simply isn't fit to count.*
>
> *"So we have great schools of medical practice, each with its well-satisfied adherents, living on in absolute ignorance of each other and of each other's experience. How many of the graduates, recent or early, of the Harvard Medical School, have spent 24 hours of their lives in experimen-*

tally testing homoeopathic remedies or seeing them tested? Probably not 10 in the whole Commonwealth . . . 'Of such experience as that,' they say, 'give me ignorance rather than knowledge.' And the club opinion of the Massachusetts Medical Society pats them on the head and backs them up . . . Even the very best type (of mind) is partly blind. There are methods which it cannot bring itself to use. The blindness of a type of mind is not diminished when those who have it band themselves together in a corporate profession. By just as much as they hold each other up to a high standard in certain lines and force each other to be thorough and conscientious there, by just so much along the other lines do they not only permit but even compel each other to be shallow. When I was a medical student, I feel sure that any one of us would have been ashamed to be caught looking into a homoeopathic book by a professor. We had to sneer at homoeopathy by word of command. Such was the school opinion at that time, and I imagine that similar encouragements to superficiality in various directions exist in the medical schools of today. . . ." [391]

According to the medical historian Harris L. Coulter, PhD, this speech was never published in any collections of James' works, even though, as he wrote to a friend, "it required the greatest moral effort of my life."[392]

For drug companies, homeopathy represents a virtual nightmare in terms of competition because it is not only very effective, it also is also extremely inexpensive. It is, literally, dirt cheap. One pellet of a properly prescribed homeopathic remedy costs only about 3 pennies and may completely and rapidly cure an acute malady such as a flu, otitis, or a food poisoning, while treating these by conventional means may require up to $50 or more in over-the-counter or prescription drugs, not counting the hundreds of dollars that might be spent on medical tests. To make matters even worse from the point of view of pharmaceutical commerce, the majority of homeopathic remedies cannot be patented. Finally, in most cases one cannot amass retail sales of many homeopathic remedies because proper prescription is not based on generic medical conditions but on strictly individualized evaluation (i.e. a group of people who suffer from the same flu, food poisoning, or strep throat may receive many different remedies, depending not so much on their generic diagnosis but on the individual way their bodies express these conditions).

Moreover, people who are successfully treated homeopathically rather than allopathically enjoy faster recovery and longer remissions, without requiring numerous doctor's visits, specialists, or interventions of any kind. Insurance companies in the later part of the 1800's recognized this and were offering discounted rates on life insurance policies to the homeopathically treated population because official statistics indicated that they were in better health and were living longer.[393]

Considering the medical economics involved, it should be obvious that homeopathy did not readily lend itself to becoming a source of profits for the pharmaceutical companies or medical establishment.

The concerns of mainstream medicine grew directly in proportion to the growing popularity of homeopathy. As expressed in the *Journal of American Medical Association: "We all know perfectly well that the sympathy of the press generally and one of the public is with the homeopaths."* [394] This statement, however, was not meant to be a pronouncement of an official surrender but rather the expression of a dire need to turn the tables around.

Even the AMA officially recognized the great conflict of interest and commercialism that was taking place in national health care at the turn of the century. In 1906, the *Journal of American Medical Association* published this statement: *"The medical press is profoundly under the influence of the proprietary interests"* (i.e. drug companies). This same medical press was brainwashing conventional physicians against homeopaths, calling them "immoral" and "illegitimate," while the AMA saw it as their duty to protect the professional and financial self-interests of their constituents. Very few are aware today that the very existence of the AMA is owed, at least partly, to the success of homeopathy in 19th century. Here is a quote from *"History of Medicine"* as taught to medical students at the present time in the U.S.:

*"For example, in the nineteenth century United States, doc-
tors resented the financial threat and personal success (as
much as they mistrusted the knowledge) of their 'unortho-
dox' colleagues, the homeopathics, eclectics, Thomsonians,
and midwives. The American Medical Association was
founded in 1847 partly as a professional lobby to protect the
market share of doctors against homeopathists."* [395]

It is of interest that orthodox medicine has never presented scientific evidence against homeopathy. Indeed, the professional allopathic organizations have purposely avoided engaging in formal trials where homeopathic medicines and the homeopathic method of
treatment could be tested. For example, in 1912 the American Institute of Homeopathy proposed that the AMA conduct controlled
clinical trials of homeopathy. This proposal was met without enthu-
siasm and the trials never occurred. [396]

On occasion, spokesmen for mainstream allopathic medicine
make claims that homeopathy has been rejected by the majority of
the medical profession because it has failed scientific investigation.
Such claims are false; no scientific investigations have been conducted whose results were detrimental to the credibility of homeopathy. [397]

Unable to defeat homeopathy on professional grounds, the medical establishment and the pharmaceutical industry has resorted to
political tactics. Regretfully, they have often been successful, to the
great detriment of the American health care system and the people.

In 1910, the Flexner Commission, headed by Senator Abram
Flexner and staffed with conventional medical experts, in cooperation with the leading members of the AMA, issued a report evaluat-
ing U.S. medical schools. Not surprisingly, the commission found
that conventional allopathic medical schools conformed to the "high
scientific standards" in offering the proper medical training,
whereas homeopathic colleges did not meet the "high criteria." The
report placed the most value on the pathological and chemical
analysis of the human body, the main target of pharmaceutical products, and discounted the value of the "rather nebulous philosophi-
cal" energetic aspects of humans emphasized in homeopathy.

Homeopathic colleges attempted to overcome the ramifications of the report and to conform to conventional standards by increasing the number of hours devoted to allopathic education at the expense of quality homeopathic training. This produced fewer capable homeopathic doctors, while newly established clauses approved by the majority of State Medical Boards made it extremely difficult for most homeopaths to practice medicine. In addition, homeopathic colleges had to incur huge expenses to acquire new teaching staff, equipment and facilities in order to meet the imposed allopathic standards of education while cutting back on expenses within their traditional curriculum.

Mr. John D. Rockefeller, Sr. was angered by this new state of affairs: ". . . My fear that injustice was being done to homeopathists . . . I would like to be more certain that the homeopathic interests are receiving fair treatment at our hands." He admonished his staff to appropriate funds on behalf of the struggling homeopathic institutions. But he was deceived by his advisors on medical matters who were under the heavy influence of the top allopath at the time, Dr. Osler, and the moneys were diverted to allopathic schools instead.[398]

Within a few years of the release of the Flexner Report in 1910, almost all of the homeopathic colleges, hospitals and pharmacies in the U.S. were out of business. Since then, homeopathy has been kept alive through the efforts of lay homeopaths.

One layman, U.S. Senator from New York, Royal Copland, was instrumental in making homeopathy a part of the Federal Food, Drug and Cosmetic Act of 1938.[399] It was based on the guidelines for homeopathic practice provided by the Homeopathic Pharmacopoeia Convention of the United States (HPCUS), an organization composed of clinicians, pharmacists and scientists with high expertise in the practice of homeopathy. For over a century, since 1898, the HPCUS has been continually publishing a compendium of homeopathic remedies of the United States. Through the efforts of Sen. Copeland, HPCUS was added to the official compendium of drugs recognized and regulated under FDA law.

Homeopathy was introduced to the United States by a Bostonian physician, Hans Burch Gram, MD in 1825. Gram received his homeopathic education while undergoing his medical training in

Denmark. Upon his return to the U.S., Gram settled in New York City where he trained several orthodox physicians who then spread homeopathy throughout the New England and mid-Western states.

Around the same era, a few German physicians, including an outstanding homeopath, Constantine Hering, MD, came to Pennsylvania and established a solid training base for homeopathy in the U.S. Due to the combined efforts of Dr. Herring's and other physicians from Boston and New York, the first medical national body, the American Institute of Homeopathy, was established in 1844. Subsequently, the Homeopathic Medical College of Pennsylvania was opened in Philadelphia. Later on, the college was renamed as Hahnemann Medical College. Both the American Institute of Homeopathy and Hahnemann Medical College are still in existence today.

There are two major factors responsible for the rebirth of homeopathy in the United States and Europe over the last two decades: 1) improved scientific methods have been able to prove the non-molecular (i.e., non-chemical) energetic nature of homeopathic medicines; 2) the health consumer has grown increasingly skeptical of the ability of conventional medicine to meet the healthcare needs of the majority of the population. In addition, medicine's innate ability to undermine health either directly through drug-induced side effects or indirectly via symptom-suppressive therapies, while either dismissing or pushing the underlying pathogenic factors deeper into the body has led to graver degenerative illnesses and has forced many to fear and avoid the hi-tech medical industry.

Our official health care statistics speak for themselves. The number of people with chronic diseases in the U.S. alone is over 100 million.[400] According to the article, "One Sick Country," based on a survey conducted by *The New England Journal of Medicine* and published in *USA Today* on June 28, 2001, as many as 80% of the American population do not enjoy good health and are either popping pills or seeing doctors regularly. Our annual health care bill represents an enormous financial burden placed on the national economy by this medical monopoly. The main partakers of an annual 1.5 trillion dollar pie—drug companies, doctors, hospitals and insurance companies—do not have any solutions besides pointing fingers at one another.[401] The great majority of the health insurance sector is relying upon advice of their "medical experts," allopathically trained doctors, while denying coverage of safer and often far more effective homeopathic and other alternative treatments. It should come as no surprise that as many as 40 million Americans can no longer afford to buy medical insurance for themselves or their families. The worst is yet to come, according to A. Reinhardt, a Princeton economist, who sees double-digit increases in health insurance premiums over the next 10 years without any relief in sight.[402] Even the mainstream American media has finally realized that high-priced, hi-tech medicine and high quality medical care are not necessarily synonymous. A recent issue of *The Wall Street Journal* accused conventional medicine of an unacceptable degree of ignorance.[403] It is only logical that great numbers of people in both the United States and Europe are turning to alternative medicine and particularly, homeopathy. This trend also has been reflected in the growing number of conventional doctors themselves turning to the study of alternative medicine.

For example, a study published in the *British Medical Journal* reported that in a survey of 100 recently graduated British physicians, as many as 80% expressed their intention to learn homeopathy, acupuncture or mind-body techniques.[404] Overall, up to 37% of British family practitioners use homeopathy. In Great Britain, visits to homeopathic physicians are increasing at the rate of 39% per year. Forty-two percent of conventional doctors referred their patients for homeopathic consultations, according to the *British Medical Journal* survey.[405] There are a total of five homeopathic hospitals in Great Britain today, several of them established by the Royal Family. These along with out-patient homeopathic clinics are part of the national health care system The British Parliament has declared homeopathy to be a *bona fide* postgraduate medical specialty.

The Royal Family have been well-known supporters and consumers of homeopathy for over 150 years. Prince Charles himself exercised leadership recently in launching his *Integrative Health Care Initiative,* the aim of which is to expand the availability of homeopathy and other complementary therapies within the UK National Health Service.[406]

Today there are more than 30 million people in Europe who receive homeopathic treatment. In the Netherlands, 47% of general practitioners use alternative medicine, mostly homeopathy.[407] In Russia, 15,000 physicians use homeopathy. Many of these are conventional medical specialists in a variety of fields: psychiatry, cardiology, neurology, ENT and ophthalmology. Homeopathy also has been gaining popularity in Austria, Greece, Israel and Italy. The Italian National Research Council sponsored a major scientific analysis of homeopathy.[408] In Belgium, France, Germany and the Netherlands, over one-third of the conventional doctors use homeopathic remedies in their practices or refer patients for homeopathic treatments.[409] As many as 70% of the French population use homeopathic medicines.[410] In the 1990's, French President Mitterand and the deans of six French medical schools demanded a greater commitment to homeopathic research.[411]

Traditionally, homeopathy has been very popular in Asia and particularly in India, where Mahatma Gandhi was one of its most ardent supporters and promoters. There are over 200 homeopathic medical schools in India, with 100,000 physicians practicing homeopathy and afforded the legal status of conventional physicians.[412] A homeopathic physician, A. U. Ramakrishnan, MD, is the personal homeopath to the President of India. Dr. Ramakrishnan has written a book about the homeopathic treatment of cancer, presenting many cases in which conventional oncological treatments failed along with stunning accounts of numerous recoveries from advanced cancers even with multiple metastases which responded to homeopathy. These patients were treated with just a few homeopathic pellets at a miniscule cost. Their recoveries were confirmed with conventional blood tests, x-rays and CAT scans. Even in terminally ill patients, fairly substantial prolongation of life, and, most importantly, superior quality of life that ended in a peaceful and humane demise, were achieved.[413]

The largest allopathic hospital in Asia, Bombay Hospital of Bombay University, employs the services of the prominent and internationally known homeopath, Farokh J. Master, MD. From his allopathic colleagues he receives difficult and challenging cases that do not yield to conventional treatments, including those of patients with cancer. The overall outcome of these cases under their joint care is far superior than when left to allopathic treatment alone.

Mother Teresa introduced homeopathy into her healing ministry for the impoverished in Calcutta, Indonesia, as far back as 1950. To this day, the ministry utilizes four homeopathic dispensaries run by the Missionary of Charity Sisters. [414]

Central and South American countries like Mexico, Brazil and Argentina have numerous homeopathic schools and research institutions. In Argentina, 2,000 doctors practice homeopathy and 3,000,000 people have used homeopathic remedies.[415] In Brazil, there are several thousand doctors who use homeopathy. Brazil also enjoys at least 10 homeopathic schools as well as several conventional medical schools that provide a curriculum on homeopathy.[416] Pharmacists in Brazil are required to receive a course on homeopathic pharmacology before graduating.

There is a surge of interest in homeopathy in Africa, Australia, Japan, New Zealand, and the former eastern block European countries. More than 10,000 medical doctors are part of the International Homeopathic Medical League.[417]

In Europe, where the European Parliament has officially recognized homeopathy, the European Union requested the European Commission to further its scientific investigation of homeopathy.[418] A group of experts were appointed to the Homeopathic Medicine Research Group (HMRG). The aim of the commission is *"to seek better ways to provide high quality medical services at low cost and that would be, at the same time, highly diversified, personalized and rapidly available."* One focus of this group is to determine whether homeopathic remedies can replace pharmacological drugs in livestock feed, in order to decrease public consumption of pharmacological residues and the development of dangerous antibiotic-resistant mutations of bacterial strains.

National health care systems in Belgium, France and Germany reimburse for homeopathic medicines under the same status as conventional medications.

A very exciting clinical research initiative was undertaken by the famous British homeopath, Jeremy Sherr, PhD, and the Dutch homeopath, Jan Scholten, MD. This research involved the clinical study of the entire periodic table of elements in an attempt to uncover the immense hidden healing properties that the individual elements harbor within their corresponding energetic structure. Dr.

Scholten published this ground-breaking medical work on behalf of
humanity in his instructive book, *Homeopathy and the Elements.*[419]

The World Health Organization has recommended that homeopathy should be integrated with conventional medicine worldwide
in order to provide a higher quality of health care.[420]

In the United States, homeopathy has yet to recover from its
demolition inflicted by the medical establishment a century ago. Yet
signs of hope are there as the public and even conventional doctors
reach out in growing numbers to explore alternatives, including homeopathy. According to a recent survey, as many as 49% of primary
care physicians, members of AMA, expressed interest in training in
homeopathy.[421] This trend, however, has not gone unnoticed by the
international pharmaceutical complex.

As recently as the spring of 2002, the distinguished members of
the American Pharmaceutical Association (APhA) gathered in
Philadelphia, where a medical school still bears the name of Samuel
Hahnemann. What was its agenda? Considering the long list of
problems that compel concern within the drug industry, it might
have been one of many. For example, they might have investigated
the presence of deadly mercury in childhood vaccines that causes
devastating physical and mental damage to American children, or
the absence of any safety studies for drugs administered to children,
or the presence of myriads of allergenic additives, food stuffs and
preservatives in children's syrups administered for seizures, allergies, and asthma. Not surprisingly, the study published in the November, 2002 issue of *Pediatrics* reported serious disabilities including birth defects and deaths among thousands of children under
the age of two who were given drugs or whose mothers took drugs
during pregnancy or lactation.

They might have exposed sham drug company advertising that
attempts to hook teens and young adults on psychotropic medications from an early age, creating the "social phobia" epidemic by
promising them every success in their social and professional life.[422]

Or they might have expressed concern over our senior citi-
zens—who have become virtual walking drug stores and can no
longer afford the fiscal burden of their prescriptions, and have to
travel to another country, like Canada, to fill them.

Perhaps they would help to excoriate the sophisticated and corrupt national network, planted by the drug companies, which dragged in doctors, hospitals and their pharmacies? This has led to outright fraud, kickbacks and bribes for which the Bush Administration passed regulations in the fall of 2002, threatening criminal punishment.[423,424]

Well, it was none of these.

The subject was its old rival—homeopathy; and its aim—to eliminate HPCUS guidelines, which are used in the United States, as well as in Canada, Asia and the European Commonwealth. Even the American Medical Association, to its credit, reaffirmed the importance of the HPCUS as recently as 1996.[425]

A century has passed since Flexner's report of 1910 is a meaningless figure on the eternal scale of human greed, but one fact is sure—credit is due the members of APhA at least for this: They know well what their real competition is.

But ultimately, homeopathy and its future in the United States will lie with the people themselves—fully informed of its wonderful benefits.

Epilogue

Evidence is compelling that homeopathy, as no other medical system, can address the foundations of any disease—the causative factors consisting of the wide variety of offending agents. Homeopathic experience over more than two centuries has documented that individual constitutional predispositions down to the genetic level are well within reach of homeopathic medicines. Where homeopathy is applied with precision and through guidance afforded by a skillful Bio-resonance diagnosis, it becomes the formidable force in medicine.

Unfortunately, American health care remains dominated by special interest groups that manipulate the political process and public opinion by over-inflating the value of allopathic medical methods to the exclusion of others. Excessive monetary subsidies are expected to overcome inadequate clinical yields. For example, a petition was introduced by New York Senator Hillary Clinton to appropriate $90 million in order to extend a study of the disabled firemen and "Ground Zero" workers. It seems obvious that mere benevolent intent behind the study cannot be sufficient to yield any meaningful clinical outcomes. It will produce, instead, a $90 million rubber stamp confirming the ultimate failure of conventional methods to aid the brave men. Likewise, the entire amount of nearly $3 billion that the Bush Administration has generously appropriated to enhance our medical preparedness for terrorist events will be spent reinforcing a system whose inherent medical limitations cannot be overcome through mere monetary "injections."

In today's reality, a handful of fanatics can inflict damage of catastrophic proportions upon large civilian populations generating casualties far in excess of the capacity of existing medical facilities.

The responsibility for medical preparedness must be shared with the people themselves. Homeopathy provides the means to accomplish this. Mass public education and training in the effective administration of the prophylactic and therapeutic measures presented in this book can successfully minimize the number of immediate and long term casualties.

The few, poorly funded and professionally oppressed departments of alternative medicine in teaching hospitals in the U.S. ought to be expanded and assume a decisive lead in training a new breed of physicians—skillful, proficient and knowledgeable in what is useful in both alternative and conventional medicine. This will also serve to end the senseless professional divisiveness in our health care for which the public pays heavy tolls in both its inferior quality and exorbitant costs.

Under the present circumstances where our government officials consider future catastrophic events to be imminent, one can hardly disagree with the statement of Congressman Dan Burton (R) of Indiana that the effectiveness of some treatments for bioterrorism are being overlooked at a time when we could ill-afford to overlook any possible options.[426] Homeopathy and the system presented here provide these options and sound solutions. Their inclusion will not only assure maximum preparedness but, as importantly, empower the people themselves.

References

1. Hahnemann, Samuel. *Organon of the Medical Art* (O'Reilly, ed., 2001).
2. Miller, James G. *Living Systems* (McGraw Hill, 1978; University Press of Colorado, 1995).
3. Pert, Candace. *Molecules of Emotion, The Science Behind Mind-Body Medicine* (Simon and Schuster, 1999).
4. Tiller, William A. *Toward a Future Medicine Based on Controlled Energy Fields* (1 (1) 5–16, Phoenix, 1977).
5. Ibarra, Raul. *Biological Rhythms of Human Being, General Bibliography* (1960–1997), San Diego, CA. 1998.
6. De Schepper, Luc. *Hahnemann Revisited, A Textbook of Classical Homeopathy for the Professional* (Full of Life Publishing, Santa Fe, 1999).
7. Bellosi, A., *et al.*, (1985) "Is there an association between myocardial infarction and geomagnetic activity?" *International Journal of Biometeriology* 29(1):1–6.
8. Chibrikin, VM, *et al.*, (1995) "Dynamics of social processes and geomagnetic activity, 1: periodic components of variations in the number of recorded crimes in Moscow." *Biofizika* 40(5):1050–1053.
9. Kay, RW (1994) "Geomagnetic storms: association with incidence of depression as measured by hospital admission." *British Journal of Psychiatry* 164(3): 403–409.
10. Stoupel, E., *et al.*, (1991) "Admissions of patients with epileptic seizures and dizziness related to geomagnetic and solar activity levels: differences in female and male patients." *Medical Hypotheses* 36(4): 384–388.
11. Stoupel, E., *et al.*, (1995) "Ambulatory blood pressure moni-

toring in patients with hypertension on days of high and low geomagnetic activity." *Journal of Human Hypertension.* 9(4):293–294.

12. Dossey, Larry. *Healing Words: The Power of Prayer and the Practice of Medicine* (Harper San Francisco, October 1997).

13. Smith, Cyril W., Best, Simon. *Electromagnetic Man—Health and Hazard in the Electrical Environment* (J.M. Dent & Sons Ltd., 1989).

14. Luu, C. *Etude des Dilutions Homeopathiques par Spectroscopie Raman-Laser, Essai d'Interpretation de Leur Mechanisme d'Action. (Ed. Boirin, Paris,* 1976).

15. Barros, J., Pasteur, St. *Omeopatia, Medicina del Terreno.* (1984) F. Palombi Editore (original edition: *Homeopatia, Medicina del Terreno* (1977), E. Bibl. Universitad Central de Venezuela, Caracas).

16. Smith, R., Boericke, G. W. (1966) "Modern instrumentation for the evaluation of homeopathic drug structure", *J. Am. Inst. Hom.* 59:263.

17. Young, T.M. (1975) "NMR studies of succussed solutions: a preliminary report." *J. Am. Inst.Hom.* 68:8.

18. Lasne, Y., *et al.,* (1989) "Contribution a l'approche scientifique de la doctrine homeopathique." *De Natura Rerum* 3: 38.

19. Smith, R. B., Boericke, G. W. (1968) "Changes caused by succussion on NMR patterns and bioassay of bradykinin triacetate succussions and dilutions." *J. Am. Inst. Hom.* 61:197–212.

20. Sachs, A.D. (1983) "Nuclear magnetic resonance spectroscopy of homeopathic remedies." *J. Holistic Med.* 5: 172–175.

21. Demangeat, S. L. *et al.,* (1992) "Modifications des temps de relaxation RMN a 4 MHz des protons du solvant dans les tres hautes dilutions salines de Silice/Lactose." *J. Med. Nucl. Biophy.* 16 (2): 135.

22. Sachs, A.D. (1983) "Nuclear magnetic resonance spectroscopy of homeopathic remedies." *J. Holistic Med.* 5: 172–175.

23. Ibid.

24. Smith C.W., Endler P.C. (1994) "Resonance phenomena of an ultra high dilution of thyroxin—preliminary results." In: Endler, P.C., Schulte, J. (Eds.) *Ultra High Dilution: Physiology and Physics.* Dordrecht: Kluwer Academic, 203–207.

25. Ludwig, W. (1986, 1988), Papers presented at seminars of the Brügemann Institute, Postfach 1262, Pippinstrasse *10,* D-8035 Gauting, W. Germany.

26. Del Giudice, E. *et al.,* (1988a) "Water as a free electric dipole laser." *Phys. Rev. Lett.* 61: 1085.

27. Endler, P. Christian, *et al.,* (Fall, 1993) "Effects of Highly Diluted Succussed Thyroxine on Amphibia Development." *The Center for Frontier Sciences,* Volume 3, Number 2.

28. Tiller, William A. *Science and Human Transformation: Subtle Energies, Intentionality and Consciousness* (Pavior Publishing, 1997).

29. Lo, SY (1996) *Modern Physics Lett.* B19:909–919.

30. Tiller, William A. *Science and Human Transformation, Subtle Energies, Intentionality and Consciousness* (Pavior Publishing, 1997).

31. Lakhovsky, G. *The Secret of Life* (Clement. M., London: Heinemann, 1939).

32. Ibid.

33. Ibid.

34. Gurwitsch A. A., (1932) "Die Mitogenetische Strahlhung des Markhaltigen Nerven," *Pflugers Arch.ges.Physiol.* vol. 231, pp.234.

35. Ostrander, S. *Psychic Discoveries Behind the Iron Curtain* (Prentice Hall, 1984).

36. Becker, Robert O., Selden, Gary. *The Body Electric, Electromagnetism and the Foundation of Life* (Morrow Publishing, 1985).

37. Crile, George. *The Phenomena of* Life. A Radio-Electric Interpretation. (William Heinemann, Ltd. Publishers, London).

38. Rapp, P.E., (1979) "An Atlas of Cellular Oscillators, Experimental Biology," *J. exp. Biol.* 81, 281–306, Great Britain.

39. Nordenström, Björn E.W. *Biologically Closed Electric Circuits: Clinical, Experimental and Theoretical Evidence for an Additional Circulatory System* (Coronet Books, January 1983).

40. Ostrander, S. *Psychic Discoveries Behind the Iron Curtain* (Prentice Hill, 1984).
41. Becker, Robert O. *Cross Currents* (G.P. Putnam's Sons, Putnam Berkley Group, Inc., 1990).
42. Tiller, William A. *Science and Human Transformation—Subtle Energies, Intentionality and Consciousness* (Pavior Publishing, 1997).
43. Tiller, William A., *et al.*, *Conscious Acts of Creation—The Emergence of a New Physics* (Pavior Publishing, 2001).
44. Smith, C.W. (1995) "Electromagnetic aspects of biological cycles." *Environmental Medicine* 9(3): 113–118.
45. Busch, H. *The Molecular Biology of Cancer* (Academic Press, New York, 1974, ed.).
46. Schroeder, G. *The Hidden Face of God.* (The Free Press, 2001).
47. Smith, Cyril W., Best, Simon. *Electromagnetic Man—Health and Hazard in the Electrical Environment* (J.M. Dent & Sons Ltd., 1989)
48. Smith, Cyril W. (Fall/Winter 1998) "Is a Living System a Macroscopic Quantum System?" *Frontier Perspectives.* Vol. 7, Number 1, p. 9–15.
49. Baumans, V., *et al.*, "Does Chelidonium 3X lower serum cholesterol? *Brit. Hom. J.*, (1987, 76, 14–15).
50. Swicord, M.L., Davis, C. C. (1983) "Bioelectromagnetics", 4(1), 21–42.
51. Kremer, F., *et al.*, (1988) "The influence of low-intensity millimeter waves on biological systems." In: *Biological Coherence and Response to External Stimuli* (H. Frohlich, ed.). Springer-Verlag, Berlin, p. 86.
52. Popp, F.A., *et al.*, (1994) "Biophoton emission: experimental background and theoretical approaches." *Modern Physics Letters B*, 8(21/22).
53. Poponin, V., *DNA and Cellular Research* (Institute of HeartMath, 1995).
54. Adey, W.R. (1988) "Physiological signaling across cell membranes and cooperative influences of extremely low frequency electromagnetic fields." In: *Biological Coherence and Response to External Stimuli.* Fröhlich H (ed) Springer-Verlag. Berlin. P. 148.

55. Del Giudice, E., *et al.*, (1998b) "Structures, correlations and electromagnetic interactions in living matter: Theory and applications." In: *Biological Coherence and Response to External Stimuli* (H. Frohlich, ed.). Springer-Verlag, Berlin, p. 49.

56. Del Giudice, E. (1990) "Collective processes in living matter: A key for homeopathy." In: *Homeopathy in Focus.* VGM (Verlag für Ganzheitsmedizin) Essen, p. 14.

57. Popp, F., *et al.,* In: *Electromagnetic Bio-Information* (Vienna: Urban & Schwarzenberg, 1989).

58. Smith, C., (1990) "Homoeopathy, structure and coherence." In: Zentrum Dokumentacion Natura Heil Kunde (ed.). *Homeopathy in Focus.* Essen: Verlag für Ganzheitsmedizin.

59. Smith, C., In: *Electromagnetic Bio-information* (Vienna: Urban & Schwarzenberg, 1989).

60. Kaznacheyev, V.P., et al., (1974) "Apparent Information Transfer Between Two Groups of Cells", *Institute of Clinical and Experimental Medicine and Institute of Automation and Electrometry, Academy of Science,* Novosibirsk, USSR.

61. Smith, C.W., *et al.,* (1985) "Water—friend or foe?" *Lab. Pract.* **34:** 29.

62. Monro, J. (1987) "Electrical sensitivities in allergic patients." *Clin. Ecol.* **4:** 93.

63. Smith, C.W., (1988) "Electromagnetic effects in humans." In: Frohlich H (ed) *Biological Coherence and Response to External Stimuli.* Springer-Verlag, Berlin, p.205.

64. Smith, C.W., (1989) "Coherent electromagnetic fields and bio-communication." In: Popp FA *et al* (eds) *Electromagnetic Bio-Information.* Urban and Swarzenberg, München, p.1.

65. Smith, C.W. (1994) "Electromagnetic and magnetic vector potential bio-information and water." In: Endler PC, Schulte, J (eds) *Ultra High Dilution.* Kluwer Acad. Publ., Dordrecht, p. 187.

66. Van Wijk, R., Schamhart, D.H., (1988) "Regulatory aspects of low intensity photon emission", *Experientia* 44, Birhäuser Verlag, CH-4010 Basel, Switzerland.

67. Iyengar, R. (1996) "Gating by cyclic AMP: Expanded role for an old signaling pathway." *Science* 271: 461–463, In: Bellavite, P, Signorini, A., *The Emerging Science of Homeopathy—Complexity, Biodynamics, Nanopharmacology* (2002), *North Atlantic Books.*

68. Mandelbrot, B.B. *The Fractal Geometry of Nature* (W.H. Freeman & Co., New York, 1982).
69. Sander, L.M. (1987) "Fractal growth." *Sci. Am.* 256 (1): 82.
70. Goldberger, A.L., *et al.*, (1990) "Chaos and fractals in human physiology." *Sci. Am.* 262 (2): 34.
71. Gutzwiller, M.C. (1992) "Quantum chaos." *Sci. Am.* 266: 26.
71a. Gardner, C., Hock, N. (1991) "Chaos Theory and Homeopathy", *Berlin J. Res. Homeopathy* 1: 236.
72. Lorenz, E.N. (1963) "Deterministic nonperiodic flow." *J. Atmos. Sci.* 20: 130–141.
73. Cramer, F. *Chaos and Order: The Complex Structure of Living Systems* (Weinheim:.VCH Verlagsgesellschaft, 1993).
74. Nugent, A.M., *et al.*, (1994) "Variable patterns of atrial natriuretic peptide secretion in man." *Eur. J. Clin. Invest.* 24: 267–274.
75. Goldberger, A.L. (1996) "Non-linear dynamics for clinicians: Chaos theory, fractals, and complexity at the bedside." *Lancet* 347: 1312–1314.
76. Freeman, W.J. (1991). "The physiology of perception." *Sci.* 264: 34–41.
77. Shinbrot, T., *et al.*, (1993) "Using small perturbations to control chaos." *Nature* 363: 411–417.
78. Lorenz, E.N. (1979) "Predictability: Does the flap of a butterfly's wings in Brazil set off a tornado in Texas?" *Address at the Annual Meeting of the American Association for the Advancement of Science,* Washington, DC.
79. *A Dictionary of Physics* (Oxford University Press, 1996).
80. Griffiths, D. *Introduction to Elementary Particles* (John Wiley & Sons, Inc. New York, 1987).
81. Tiller, William A. *Science and Human Transformation: Subtle Energies, Intentionality and Consciousness* (Pavior Publishing, 1997).
82. Nobili, R. (1987) "Ionic Waves in Animal Tissues." *Physical Reviews A* 35-1901–22.
83. (Lo, SY *et al.*, (1996) "Physical Properties of Water with I_E Structures." *Modern Physics Letters* **B10:** 921–930.
84. Lo, SY. (1996) *Modern Physics Lett.* **B19:** 909–919.
85. Lo, SY. Bonavida, B. *Proceedings of the First International*

Symposium on Physical, Chemical and Biological Properties of Stable Water [I_E] Clusters. (Singapore: World Scientific Publishing, 1998).

86. Hartmann, Franz, *Life and the Doctrines of Philippus Theophrastus Bombast of Hohenheim Known as Paracelsus* (Kessinger Publishing Company, October 1998).

87. Heiby, Walter, *The Reverse Effect* (MediScience Publishers, 1988).

88. Luckey, T.D. (1999). "Nurture with ionizing radiation: a provocative hypothesis." *Nutr. Cancer* 34: 1–11.

89. Richet, C., (1905) *Archs. Int. Physio.*, 3 (1905) 203.

90. Richet, C., (1906) *Archs. Int. Physio.*, 3 (1906) 264.

91. Richet, C., (1906) *Archs. Int. Physio.*, 4 (1906) 18.

92. Hotchkiss, M., Bacteriol.,J., 8 (1923) 141.

93. Miller, W.S., *et al.*, *Nature,* London, 155 (1945) 210.

94. Pratt, R., and Dufrenoy, J., *Bacteriol. Rev.*, 12 (1948) 79.

95. Randall, W.A., *et al.*, *Am. J. Publ. Health,* 37 (1947) 421.

96. Loefer, J.B., *et al.*, *Bull. Torrey Bot. Club,* 79 (1952) 242.

97. Goldstein, S., *Science,* 84 (1936) 176.

98. Dunstan, W.M., *et al.*, *Mar. Biol.*, 31 (1975) 305.

99. Prouse, N.J., *et al.*, *J. Fish. Res. Bd. Can.*, 33 (1975) 810.

100. Jennings, J.R., *J. Plankt. Res.*, 1 (1979) 121.

101. Mottram, J.C., *Nature,* London., 144 (1939) 154.

102. Gabliks, J., *Proc. Soc. Exp. Biol. Med.*, 120 (1965) 168.

103. Gabliks, J., *et al.*, *Proc. Soc. Exp. Biol. Med.*, 125 (1967) 1002.

104. Browne, C.L., and Davis, L.E., *Cell Tissue Res.*, 177 (1977) 555.

105. Reish, D.J., and Carr, R.S., *Mar. Pollut. Bull.*, 9 (1978) 24.

106. Engel, D.W., and Davis, E.M. in Cushing, C. E. (Ed.), *Radioecology and Energy Resources* (Dowden, Hutchinson & Ross, Stroudsberg, 1976).

107. Engel, D.W., *Radiat. Res.*, 32 (1967) 685.

108. Weis, J.S., and Mantel, L.H., *Estuarine Coastal Mar. Sci.*, 4 (1976) 461.

109. Luckey, T.D., *J. Econ. Entomol.*, 61 (1968) 7.

110. Leduc, G., *J. Fish. Res. Bd. Can.*, 35 (1978) 166.

111. Gruger, E.H., *et al.*, *Environ. Sci. Technol.*, 10 (1976) 1033.

112. Luckey, T.D., In: *Proceedings First International Conference on the Use of Antibiotics in Agriculture* (1956), NAS-NRC Publ. No. 397, Washington.
113. Morehouse, N.F., *Poultry Sci.*, 28 (1949) 375.
114. Stare, F.J., *Nutr. Rev.*, 14 (1956) 206.
115. Smyth, H.F., *et al.*, *J. Ind. Hyg. Toxicol.*, 18 (1936) 277.
116. Lorenz, E., *et al.*, in R. E. Zirkle (Ed.), *Biological Effects of External X and Gamma Radiation* (McGraw-Hill, New York, 1954).
117. Neafsey, Patricia J., "Longevity Hormesis. A Review." *Mechanisms of Aging and Development*, 51 (1990) 1–31.
118. Weiner, H.L., *et al.*, (1994) "Oral tolerance: Immunologic mechanisms and treatment of animal and human organ-specific autoimmune diseases by oral administration of autoantigens." *Annu. Rev. Immunol.* 12: 809–837.
119. Weiner, H.L. (1997). "Oral tolerance: Immune mechanisms and treatment of autoimmune diseases." *Immunol. Today* 7: 336–343.
120. Heine, H., Schmolz, M. (2000). "Immunoregulation via 'bystander suppression' needs minute amounts of substances—a basis for homeopathic therapy?" *Med. Hypotheses* 54: 392–393.
121. Bellavite, P., *et al.*, (1997). "Scientific reappraisal of the 'Principle of Similarity'." *Med. Hypoth.* 49: 203–212.
122. Stebbing, A.R.D. *Hormesis—The Stimulation of Growth by Low Levels of Inhibitors, The Science of the Total Environment* (Elsevier Scientific Publishing Company, Amsterdam—Printed in the Netherlands, 22 (1982) 213–234).
123. Smyth, H. F., Jr. Ed. *Sufficient Challenge* (Cosmet. Toxicol. Vol. 5. p. 51–58, Pergamon Press, 1967).
124. Speech at the British Pharmaceutical Conference (1981).
125. Steinbach, D., (1981), "The Pros and Cons of Homeopathy." *Pharmaceutical Journal*, 227:384–387.
126. Kuhn, Thomas S. *The Structure of Scientific Revolutions*, Third Edition (The University of Chicago Press, 1996).
127. Taubes, Gary. (July 7, 2002) "What if it's all been a big fat lie? *The New York Times Magazine*.
128. Kleinfeld, Sonny. *The Machine Called Indomitable* (Times Books, 1986).

129. Becker, Robert O., Selden, Gary, *The Body Electric, Electromagnetism and the Foundation of Life* (Morrow Publishing, 1985).

130. Ibid.

131. Calabrese, Edward J., "Expanding the Reference Dose Concept to Incorporate and Optimize Beneficial Effects While Preventing Toxic Responses from Nonessential Toxicants", Regulatory Toxicology and Pharmacology 24, S68–S75 (1996), Article No. 0080, University of Massachusetts.

132. Hively, Will., (December 2002) "Is Radiation Good for You?" Discover, Vol. 23, No. 12.

133. Ottoboni, M. Alice, *The Dose Makes the Poison* (Vincente Books, Berkley, Ca, 1984).

134. Calabrese, Edward J., *et al.,* (1987) *"The Occurrence of Chemically Induced Hormesis",* Health Physics Vol. 52, No. 5 (May) pp. 531–541.

135. Linde, Klaus, *et al.,* (July,1994)"Critical Review and Meta-Analysis of Serial Agitated Dilutions in Experimental Toxicology," *Hum Exp Toxicol;* 13(7):481–92; Projekt Munchener Modell, Ludwig-Maximilians-Universitat, Munchen, GFR.

136. Kleijnen, *et al.,* (1991) "Clinical Trials of Homeopathy." *British Medical Journal* 302: 316–323.

137. "Homeopathy much ado about nothing" (March, 1994) *Consumer Reports.*

138. "Americans lag in science literacy", (May 1, 2002) *USA Today.*

139. Schroeder, G., *The Hidden Face of God* (The Free Press, 2001).

140. Davidson, Jonathan RT, *et al.,* (January 1997) "Homeopathic Treatment of Depression and Anxiety, Alternative Therapies." Vol. 3, No. 1.

141. Kleijnen, *et al.,* (1991) "Clinical trials of homeopathy." *BMJ;* 302: 316–323.

142. Linde, Klaus *et al.,* (1997) "Are the clinical effects of homeopathy placebo effects ?, A meta-analysis of placebo-controlled trials." *Lancet,* 350: 834–43.

143. Gell-Mann, Murray, *Quark and a Jaguar* (W.H. Freeman and Company, New York, 1994).

144. Ibid.

145. Schrödinger, Erwin (April, 1992). "What is Life?: The Physical Aspect of the Living Cell with Mind and Matter and Autobiographical Sketches." *Press Syndicate of the University of Cambridge.*

146. Peliti, L., *Biologically Inspired Physics* (Plenum Press, New York, 1991).

147. Tiller, W. A., (1977) "Toward a Future Medicine Based on Controlled Energy Fields", *Phoenix* 1 (1), 5–16.

148. Miller, James G. *Living Systems* (McGraw Hill, 1978); (University Press of Colorado, 1995).

149. Knox, S., (Spring 2000) "Physics, Biology and Acupuncture: Exploring the Interface.", *Frontier Perspectives* vol. 9 #1.

150. Ramakrishnan, A.U., Coulter, Catherine R., *A Homeopathic Approach to Cancer* (Quality Medical Publishing, 2001, p.18).

151. Ibid, p. 19.

152. "A Piece of My Mind" (February 27, 1991) *Journal of the American Medical Association.*

153. National Research Council, Washington, DC.

154. Black, F. (1843). "On the preservative properties of belladonna in scarlet fever", British *Journal of Homeopathy* 1:129–141.

155. Coulter, Harris L., *Divided Legacy: The Conflict Between Homoeopathy and the American Medical Association* (North Atlantic Books, 1973, 1982).

156. Kayne, Steven, *Homeopathic Pharmacy* (Churchill Livingstone, 1997).

157. Ullman, D., *Homeopathy: Medicine for the 21st Century* (North Atlantic Books, Berkeley, 1991a).

158. Bradford, Thomas L. *The Logic of Figures or Comparative Results of Homoeopathic and Other Treatments* (Philadelphia: Boericke and Tafel, 1900, p. 68).

159. Coulter, Harris L. *Divided Legacy: The Conflict Between Homoeopathy and the American Medical Association* (North Atlantic Books, 1973, 1982).

160. Ibid.

161. Traub, M., (Dec 2001) *Homeopathic prophylaxis: Synopsis of published research.* Homeopathy Today, Volume 21, Number 11)

162. Murphy, R., *Lotus Materia Medica* (Lotus Star Academy, 1995).
163. Currim, Ahmed, *The Collected Works of Arthur Hill Grimmer M.D.,* (Hahnemann International Institute for Homeopathic Documentation, 1996).
164. Eizayaga, F., (1985) "Tratamiento Homeopatico de las enfermedades agudas y su prevension." *Homeopatia,* V. 51, No. 342, p. 352–362.
165. Eisfelder, H.W., (Nov–Dec 1961) "Poliomyelitis Immunization: A Final Report." *Journal of the American Institute of Homeopathy,* Vol. 54, , 166–167.
166. Castro, D., Nogueira, C.G., (1975) "Use of the nosode Meningococcinum as a preventive against meningitis." *Journal of the American Institute of Homeopathy,* V.68, 211–219.
167. Eizayaga, F., (1985) "Tratamiento Homeopatico de las enfermedades agudas y su prevension." *Homeopatia,* V. 51, No. 342, p. 352–362.
168. Jonas, W.B., *et* al, (1991) "Prophylaxis of tularemia infection in mice using agitated ultra-high dilutions of tularemia-infected tissue." In:proc. 5th GIRI Meeting, Paris, Albs. 21.
169. Chavanon, P., *La Diphterie* (1932), 4e edl, Imprimerrie St-Denis, Niort.
170. Paterson, J. & Boyd, W.E., (1941) "Potency Action: A Preliminary Study of the Alteration of the Schick Test by a Homeopathic Potency," *British Homeopathic Journal,* V.31, 301–309.
171. Eizayaga, F., (1985) "Tratamiento Homeopatico de las enfermedades agudas y su prevension." *Homeopatia,* V. 51, No. 342, p. 352–362.
172. Van Erp, V.M.A., and Brands, M., (1996) "Homeopathic Treatment of Malaria in Ghana." *Brit. Homeop-J,* vol.85 pp. 66–70.
173. Golden, Isaac (1997) Aurum Pty, Ltd. Australia.
174. Marichal, B.J., Jenaer, M.C. (1990) "Immunotherapy at infinitesimal doses." *Int. Congress on Ultralow doses,* Univ. Of Borduaux.
175. "From Neuroscience to Naturopathy" (1996), *Alternative Therapies in Health and Medicine;* 2.5:80–89.
176. Tobin, Steven, *Homeopathy Today,* Sept. 1994.

177. Bradford, Thomas L. *The Logic of Figures or Comparative Results of Homoeopathic and Other Treatments* (Philadelphia,: Boericke and Tafel, 1900).

178. Lapp, C., *et al.,* (1955) "Mobilization de l'arsenic fixé chez le cobaye sous l'influence des doses infinitesimales d'arseniate." *Therapie* 10: 625.

179. Wurmser, L., Ney, J., (1955) "Mobilisation de l'arsenic fixé chez le cobaye, sous l'action de doses infinitesimales d'arseniate de sodium." *Therapie* 10:625.

180. Cazin, J.C., *et al.,* (1987) "A study of the effect of decimal and centesimal dilutions of Arsenic on the retention and mobilization of Arsenic in the rat." *Human Toxicology* 6: 315.

181. Cazin, J.C., *et al.,* (1991) "Influence of several physical factors on the activity of ultra low doses." In: *Ultra Low Doses* (C. Doutremepuich, ed.). Taylor and Francis, London, p. 69.

182. Herkovits, Perez-Coll C., Zeni W. (1988) "Reduced toxic effect of Cd on bufo arenarum embryos by means of very diluted and stirred solutions of Cd." *Communicationes Biologicas;*7:70–73.

183. (Delbancut, A., *et al.,* (1993) "Protective effect of very low concentrations of heavy metals (cadmium and cisplatin) against cytotoxic doses of these metals on renal tubular cell cultures." *Brit. Hom J.* 82: 123.

184. Fisher, P., Capel, I.D. (1982) "The treatment of experimental lead intoxication in rats by plumbum metallicum und penicillamine." *Proceedings of the 35th Congress of the Liga Medicorum Homoeopathica Internationis,* London: 320–332.

185. Fisher, P. *et al.,* "The influence of the homeopathic remedy *plumbum metallicum* on the excretion kinetics of lead in rats." *Human Toxicol. 6: 321I.*

186. Projetti, M.L., *et al.,*(1985) "Effets curatifs et préventifs de dilutions homéopatiques de sulfate de cuivre appliquées à des racines de lentilles pré- ou post-intoxiquées." *Cahiers de Biothérapie;* 88:21–27.

187. Cambar, J., *et al.,* (1983) "Mise en évidence de l'effet protecteur de dilutions homéopathiques de Mercurius corrosivus vis-à-vis de la mortalité au chlorure mercurique chez la souris." *Ann Hom. Fr.* 25 (5): 160.

188. Guillemain, *et al.*, (1984) "Effet protecteur de dilutions homéopathiques de metaux néphrotoxiques vis-à-vis d'une intoxication mercurielle." *Cah. Biothérapie* 81 (suppl.): 27.

189. Boirin J., Marin J., (1965 a & b) "Action de dilutions successives de $HgCl_2$ sur la respiration de coléoptiles de blé." *Ann Hom Fra;* 7,259–264&635–638.

190. Blostin, R. (1990) "Arsenicum album and neurotoxic poisoning in dogs." *Proceedings of the second International Congress for Veterinary Homeopathy.* I.A.V.H., Zutphen, The Netherlands.

191. Aubin, M., *et al.*, (1980) "Etude de l'activité hépatoprotectrice de Phosphorus sur des fragments de foies des rats adultes placés en culture organotypique sur milieu artificiel après intoxication par CCl_4." *Ann Hom Fra;* 22,3,25–33.

192. Bildet J., *et al.*, (1984a) "Résistance de la cellule hépatique du rat après une intoxication infinitésimale au tétrachlorure de carbone." *Hom Fra;* 72,175–181.

193. Bildet, J., *et al.*, (1975) "Etude de l'action de differentes diluitions de Phosphorus sur l'hepatite toxique du rat." *Ann Hom. Fr.* 17 (4): 425.

194. Bildet, J., *et al.*, (1984a) "Etude au microscope électronique de l'action de diluitions de phosporus 15 CH sur l'hepatite toxique du rat." *Homéopathie Francaise* 72:211.

195. Bildet, J., *et al.*, (1984b) "Resistance de la cellule hepatique du rat aprés une intoxication infinitésimale au tetrachlorure de carbone." *Homéopathie Francaise* 72: 175.

196. Ugazio, G., *et al,* (1972) "Mechanism of protection against carbon tetrachloride by prior carbon tetrachloride administration." *Exp. Mol. Path.* 16: 281.

197. Pound, A.W., *et al,* (1973) "Decreased toxicity of DMN in rats after treatment with carbon tetrachloride." *Pathology* 5 : 233.

198. Cier, A., *et al.*, (1966) "Sur le traitement du diabéte expérimental par des dilutions infinitésimales d;alloxane." *Ann Hom. Fr.* 8:137.

199. De Gerlache, J., Lans, M. (1991) "Modulation of experimental rat liver carcinogens by ultra low doses of the carcinogens." In: *Ultra Low Doses* (C. Doutremepuich, ed.) Taylor and Francis, London, p. 17.

200. Gardes, E. (1989) "Effet d'une dilution infintésimale d'acide nalidixique sur l'élimination de cette meme molecule chez l'homme sain. Diplôme Pharmacie." *Annales Homéopathiques Franáaises;* 77(5):60.

201. Delbancut, A., *et al.*, (1993) "Protective effect of very low concentrations of heavy metals (cadmium and cisplatin) against cytotoxic doses of these metals on renal tubular cell cultures." *Brit. Hom. J.* 82: 123.

202. Guillemain, J., *et al.*, (1987) "Pharmacologie de l'infinitésimal. Application aux dilutions homéopathiques." *Homéopathie* 4: 35.

203. Pennec, J.P., Aubin, M. (1984) "Effect of Aconitum and Veratrum on the isolated perfused heart of the common heel (Anguilla-anguilla)." *Comp. Biochem. Physiol.* 776: 367.

204. Paterson J., (1944). "Report on Mustard Gas Experiments" (Glasgow & London). *J Am Inst Hom;*37:47–88.

205. Khuda-Bukhsh, A.R., Banik, S. (1991) "Assessment of cytogenetic damage in X-irradiated mice and its alteration by oral administration of potentized homeopathic drug, Ginseng D200." *Berlin J. Res. Homeopathy* 1 (4/5): 254.

206. Khuda-Bukhsh, A.R., Maity, S. (1991) "Alterations of cytogenetic effects by oral administration of a homeopathic drug, Ruta graveolens, in mice exposed to sub-lethal X-irradiation." *Berlin J. Res. Homeopathy* 1 (4/5): 264.

207. Labonia, W. *et al.*, (1986) "Acao das doses minimas na protecao do enevenamento oficido de animals de laboratorio." *Congress of Liga Medicorum Homoeopathicorum Internationalis,* Rio De Janeiro.

208. Magro, Souza I.A. *et al.*, (1986) "Reducao da nefrotoxidade induzida por aminoglucosideos." 41. *Liga Medicorum Homoeopathicorum Internationalis* Congress, Rio de Janeiro.

209. Linde, K., Jonas, W.B., *et al.*, (Jul 1994) "Critical Review and Meta-Analysis of Serial Agitated Dilutions in Experimental Toxicology." *Hum Exp Toxicol;* 13(7):481–92; Projekt Munchener Modell, Ludwig-Maximilians-Universitat, Munchen, GFR.

210. Lauppert, E., Endler, C., (1996) "Enhanced inversion effect of thyroxine 10e-10—10e-13 by agitation." Angenommen für:

Taddei-Ferretti C (Hrsg.): High Dilution Effects on Cells and Integrated Systems. Singapore: World Scientific.

211. Conforti, A., *et al.*, (1993) "Effects of high dilutions of histamine and other natural compounds on acute inflammation in rats." In: *Omeomed92* (C. Bornoroni, ed.). Editrice Compositori, Bologna, p. 163.

212. Doutremepuich, C., *et al.*, (1990) "Aspirin at very low dosage in healthy volunteers; effects on bleeding time, platelet aggregation and coagulation." *Haemostasis* 20: 99.

213. Baumans, V., *et al.*, (1987) "Does Chelidonium 3x lower serum cholesterol?" *Brit. Hom.J.*; 76,14–15.

214. Sukul, N.C., *et al.*, (1986) "Prolonged cataleptogenic effects of potentized homoeopathic drugs." *Psychopharmacology* 89: 338.

215. Sukul, N.C., (1990) "Increase in serotonin and dopamine metabilites in mouse hypothalamus following oral administration of *Agaricus muscarous* 12, a homoeopathic drug." *Science and Culture* 56: 134.

216. Sukul, N.C., *et al.*, (1991) "Neuronal activity in the lateral hypothalamus of the cat and the medial frontal cortex of the rat in response to homoeopathic drugs." *Indian Biologist* 23 (2): 17.

217. Sukul, N.C., *et al.*, (1993) "Hypothalamic neuronal responses of rats to homoeopathic drugs." In: *Omeomed 92* (C. Bornoroni, ed.). Editrice Compositori, Bologna, p. 1.

218. Angelidis, C.E., *et al.*, (1991) "Constitutive expression of heat-shock protein 70 in mammalian cells confers thermoresistance." *Eur J. Biochem. 199*, 35–39.

219. Doucet-Jaboeuf *et al.*, (1982) "Evaluation de la dose limite d'activite du facteur thymique serique." *C.R. Acad. Sc. Paris* 295:283.

220. Doucet-Jaboeuf, *et al.*, (1984) "Seasonal variations in the humoral immune response in mice following administration of thymic hormones." In: *Ann. Rev. Chronopharmacology*. Vol. 1. (A. Reinberg et al., eds.) Pergamon Press, Oxford, p. 231.

221. Doucet-Jaboeuf, *et al.*, (1985) "Actions of very low doses of biological immunomodulators on the humoral immune response in mice." *Int. J. Immunoparmacol.* 7:312.

222. Bastide, M., *et al.*, (1985) "Activity and chronopharmacology of very low doses of thymulin in mice." *Int. J. Immunotherapy* 3:191.

223. Bastide, M., *et al.*, (1987) "Immunomodulatory activity of very low doses of thymulin in mice." *Int. J. Immunotherapy* 3:191.

224. Guillemain, J., *et al.*, (1987) "Pharmacologie de l'infinitesimal. Application aux dilutions homeopathiques." *Homeopathie* 4:35.

225. Daurat, V., *et al.*, (1988) "Immunomodulatory activity of low doses of interferon a, b in mice." *Biomed & Pharmacother,* 42:197.

226. Davenas, E., (1987) "Effect on mouse peritoneal macrophages of orally administered very high dilutions of silica." *Eur. J. Pharmacol.* 135: 313.

227. Oberbaum, M., *et al.*, (1992) "Wound healing by homoeopathic Silicea dilutions in mice." *Harefuah (J. Israel Med. Ass.)* 123: 78.

228. Youbicier-Simo, B.J., *et al.*, (1993) "Effects of embrionic bursectomy and in ovo administration of highly diluted bursin on adenocorticotropic and immune responses of chickens." *Int. J. Immunother.* 9: 169.

229. Bastide, M. (1994) "Immunological examples on ultra high dilution research." In: *Ultra High Dilution* (P.C. Endler and J. Schulte, eds.). Kluwer Acad. Publ., Dordrecht, p. 27.

230. Youbicier-Simo BJ, *et al.*, (1996b) "Specific abolition reversal of pituitary-adrenal activity and control of the humoral immunity in bursectomized chickens through highly dilute bursin." *Intern. J. Immunopathol. Pharmacol.*, 9: 43–51.

231. Davenas, E., *et al.*, (30 June 1988) "Human basophil degranulation triggered by very dilute antiserum against IGE." *Nature,* Vol. 333.

232. Wilson, Cynthia, *Chemical Exposure and Human Health* (McFarland & Company, Inc. Publ., 1993)

233. U.S. General Accounting Office (June 1992), "Toxic Substances: Advantages of and Barriers to Reducing Toxic Chemicals,", Report No. GAO/RECD-92-212.

234. Casarett and Doull, *Toxicology The Basic Science of Poisons* (Klaussen, Curtis., Fifth edition. McGraw-Hill, 1996).

235. Wilson, Cynthia, (1994) "The Human Consequences of the Chemical Problem", Environmental Access Research Network.

236. Penn, I. (1982) "The Occurrence of Cancer In Immune Deficiencies" curr. probl; Cancer, 6(10): 1–64.

237. Dean, S.H., *et al.*, (1984): "Toxic modifications of the immune system", in "Toxicology: the basic science of poisons", by J. Doull; C.D. Klaussen, and M.O. Amdur. 3rd edition.

238. National Research Council, Commission on Life Sciences, Board on Environmental Studies and Toxicology, Committee on Biological Markers, Subcommittee on Immunotoxicology "Biological Markers in Immunotoxicology, " (Washington, D.C. National Academy Press).

239. Sigel, Helmut (1980) *Metal Ions in Biological Systems* vol.10. Carcinogenicity and metal Ions p.321 Astrid Sigel (Editor).

240. Gilboun, M.V. (1967) "Carcinogens, enzymes induction, and gene action" Adv. Cancer Res. 10:1–81.

241. Institute of Medicine, Division of Health Promotion and Disease Prevention. *Role of the Primary Care Physician in Occupational and Environmental Medicine.* (Washington, DC: National Academy Press, 1988).

242. Institute of Medicine, Division of Health Promotion and Disease Prevention. *Addressing the Physician Shortage in Occupational and Environmental Medicine.* (Washington D.C.: National Academy Press, 1991).

243. Chang, Louis, W., *Toxicology of Metals* (CRC Press, Inc., 1996).

244. Wilson, Cynthia. *Chemical Exposure and Human Health* (McFarland & Company, Inc. Publ., 1993)

245. Rea, William J. *Chemical Sensitivity* (vol. I, II, III, IV, CRC Press, Inc., 1992).

246. Ashford, Nicholas A., Miller, Claudia S. *Chemical Exposures Low Levels and High Stakes* (John Wiley & Sons, Inc., 1998)

247. Dean, J., *et al.*, *Immunotoxicology and Immunopharmacology* (Raven Press, NY, 1985).

248. Casarett and Doull. *Toxicology The Basic Science of Poisons* (Klaussen, Curtis, Fifth edition. McGraw-Hill, 1996).

249. Chang, Louis W. *Toxicology of Metals* (CRC Press, Inc., 1996).

250. U.S. General Accounting Office (June 1992) "Toxic Substances: Advantages of and Barriers to Reducing Toxic Chemicals," Report No. GAO/RECD-92-212.

251. Institute of Medicine, Division of Health Promotion and Disease Prevention. *Role of the primary care physician in occupational and environmental medicine.* (Washington DC: National Academy Press, 1988)

252. Institute of Medicine, Division of Health Promotion and Disease Prevention, *Addressing the Physician Shortage in Occupational and Environmental Medicine.* (Washington D.C.: National Academy Press, 1991).

253. Chang, Louis, W., "Toxicology of Metals" (1996) CRC Press, Inc.)

254. Stanway, Andrew. *Alternative Medicine—A Guide to Natural Therapies* (Penguin Books, 1979).

255. Russell, Edward W., (1973) "Report on Radionics", Suffolk, England: Neville Sperman.

256. Stearns, Guy Beckley, (Nov 15, 1932) "Body-Reflexes as a Means of Selecting a Remedy." *The Homoeopathic Recorder,* Volume XLVII, Derby, Conn., No. 11.

257. Burr, H.S., Northrop, F.S., (1935) "The Electromagnetic Field Theory," Quarterly Rev. Biol., 10:322–33.

258. Proceedings of the National Academy of Sciences, (1939) "Evidence for the existence of an Electro-Dynamic Field in Living Organisms", 25:284.

259. Northrop, F.S.C., (1931) Science and First Principles, New York, Chapters III–V.

260. "The History of Modern Physics in Its Bearing Upon Biology and Medicine", *Yale Journal of Biology and Medicine,* 1938, 10:209,227.

261. Burr, H.S. and Lane, C.T., (1935) "Electrical Characteristics of Living Systems. *Yale Journal of Biology and Medicine,* 8:31–35.

262. Burr, H.S. (March, 1947) "Field Theory in Biology." *Scientific Monthly,* Vol. LXIV. No.3, 217–225.

263. Crile, George, *The Phenomena of Life*. A Radio-Electric Interpretation. (William Heinemann, Ltd. Publishers, London).

264. Crile, J.W., (Oct. 1933) in a speech at the Congress of American College of Surgeons, Chicago.

265. Becker, Robert O., *Cross Currents* (1990) G.P. Putnam's Sons, Putnam Berkley Group, Inc.

266. Libet, B., (March–April 1989) "The Sciences" (New York Academy of Science),: 32

267. Hunt, Valerie *Infinite Mind: Science of Human Vibrations of Consciousness* (Malibu Publishing Company, 1996)

268. Chen, Kuo-Gen, (May/June 1996) "Electrical Properties of Meridians" *IEEE Engineering in Medicine and Biology*).

269. Leonhardt, H., (1980) "Fundamentals of Electracupuncture According to Voll.", Medizinisch Literarische Verlags Gesellschatmbh.Uellen.

270. Nukatani, Y. (1956) "Skin Electric Resistance, Ryo Do Raku., J., *Autonomic Nerve* 6:52.

271. Kendall, H., Kendall, F. *Muscle Testing and Function* (Baltimore: Williams and Wilkins, 1971).

272. Goodheart, G. *Applied Kinesiology,* 12th ed. (Detroit: Privately Published, 1976).

273. Mann, F. *The Meridians of Acupuncture* (London: William Heinemann Medical Books Limited, 1974).

274. Chen, Kuo-Gen, (May/June, 1996) "Applying Quantum Interference to EDST (ElectroDermal Screening Testing) Medicine Testing." *IEEE Engineering in Medicine and Biology*)

275. Tiller, W. A. *Subtle Energies in Energy Medicine.* (Frontier Perspectives, Spring 1995).

276. Becker, Robert O. *Cross Currents, The Perils of Electropollution* (St. Martin's Press, 1990).

277. Mendel, Donald. *The Myth of Neuropsychiatry: A Look at Paradoxes, Physics, and the Human Brain* (Plenum Press, 1994).

278. Talbot, Michael. *The Holographic Universe* (Harper Collins Publishers, 1991).

279. Pribram, Karl H. *Brain and Perception* (Lawrence Eribaum Associates, Inc., 1991)

280. Pert, Candace. *Molecules of Emotion, The Science Behind Mind-Body Medicine* (Simon and Schuster, 1999).

281. Sylvia, Clare. *A Change of Heart* (Little Brown and Company Publishers, 1997).

282. Voll, Reinhold, (March 1975) "Twenty Years of Electroacupuncture Diagnosis in Germany. A Progress Report." *American Journal of Acupuncture,* Vol. 3, No. 1.

283. Tsuei, JJ, Lam, F. Jr., (1983) "Case findings from a family practitioner's office using electroacupuncture according to Voll." *Am J Acupunct* 11:23–9.

284. Tsuei, JJ, *et al.*, (March, 1989.) "Study of pesticide residues in the bodies of workers at a chemical factory by Bio-resonance measurements." *R.O.C. National Science Council Reports.*

285. Tsuei JJ, Chun C., (March, 1989) "Controlled study of diabetes mellitus by bioenergetic measurement." *R.O.C. National Science Council Reports.*

286. Tsuei JJ, *et al.*, (1989) "Studies in bioenergetic correlations— study on bioenergy in diabetes mellitus patients." *Am J Acupunct* 17:31–8.

287. Tsuei JJ, *et al.*, (November 1993) "The study of bioenergetic screening model for hypertension." *R.O.C. National Science Council Reports.*

288. Chou P, *et al.*, (1995) "Clinical application of bioenergy in the cardiovascular system." Report to the *ROC National Research Institute of Chinese Medicine,* NRICM-84-103.

289. Maiwald, Med. L. (1988) "Electro-Acupuncture as a Screening Method Compared With Conventional Diagnosis and Therapy." *Biological Therapy* Vol. VI #3.

290. Voll, Reinhold, (April–June 1980), "The Phenomenon of Medicine Testing in Electroacupuncture According to Voll." *Am. J. Acupuncture,* Vol 8, No. 2.

291. Shmitt, Walter H., Jr., Leisman, Gerry. (1998) "Correlation of Applied Kinesiology muscle testing findings with serum immunoglobulin levels for food allergies." *Intern. J. Neuroscience,* Vol. 96-pp. 237–244.

292. Monti, Daniel A., *et al.*,(1999) "Muscle Test Comparisons of Congruent and Incongruent Self-Referential Statements. *Perceptual and Motor Skills,* 88, 1019–1028.

293. Levenson, R.W., *et al.*, (1990) "Voluntary facial action generates emotion-specific autonomic nervous system activity." *Psychophysiology,* 27, 363–384.

294. Pennebaker, J.W., *et al.*, "The psychophysiology of confession: linking inhibitory and psychosomatic processes." *Journal of Personality and Social Psychology,* 52, 781–793.

295. Bradley, M.M, *et al.*, (1996) "Picture media and emotions: ef-

fects of a sustained affective context." *Psychophysiology*, 33, 662–670.

296. Hawkins, David R. *Power vs. Force* (Veritas Publishing, 1995).

297. Diamond, John. *Behavioral Kinesiology* (Harper & Row, New York, 1979).

298. Citro, M., *et al.*, (1993) "Transmission of hormone signals by electronic circuitry." In: *Science Innovation 93, Meeting of the American Association for the Advancement of Science*, Boston.

299. Citro, M., *et al*, (1994) "Transfer of information from molecules by means of electronic amplification. Preliminary studies." In: *Ultra High Dilution* (P.C. Endler and J. Schulte, eds.). Kluwer Acad. Publ., Dordrecht, p. 209.

300. Aissa, J., *et al.*, (1993) "Transfer of molecular signals via electronic circuitry." *FASEB J.* 7: A602 (3489).

301. Benveniste J., *et al.*, (1994b) "Transfer of the molecular signal by electronic amplification." *FASEB J.* 8 (4): Abs. 2304).

302. Endler, P.C., *et al.*,(1995) "Non-molecular information transfer from thyroxine to frogs with regard to 'homoepathic' toxicology." *J Vet & Human Toxicol*, 37 (3).

303. Thomas, Y., *et al.*, (1995) "Direct transmission to cells of a molecular signal (phorbol myristate acetate, PMA) via an electronic device." FASEB J. ;9 in press (Abs).

304. Smith, Cyril W., Best, Simon. *Electromagnetic Man—Health and Hazard in the Electrical Environment* (J.M. Dent & Sons Ltd., 1989)

305. Seneskowitsch, F., *et al.*,(1995) "Hormone effects by CD record.reply." *FASEB J.* :9 (Abs. 12161).

306. "Terrorism with Ionizing Radiation", General Guidance, the Employee Education System for the Office of Public Health and Environmental Hazards. Dept. of Veteran Affairs.

307. "Home Preparation Procedure for Emergency Administration of Potassium Iodide Tablets to Infants and Small Children." U.S. Food and Drug Administration, Center for Drug Evaluation and Research.

308. Kircher: *Mundus Subterranius*. (Amsterdam, 1645).

309. Fludd, Robert. *Philosophia Myosaica Goudae*, 1638.

310. Julian, O.A. *Materia Medica of Nosodes with Repertory* (B. Jain publishers (P), Ltd., 1996)

311. Allen, H.C. *Allen's Key Notes with Nosodes* (B. Jain Publishers Pvt. Ltd., 1990)

312. Bellavite, P., *et al.,* (1997). "Scientific reappraisal of the 'Principle of Similarity.'" *Med. Hypoth.* 49: 517–541.

313. Weiner, H.L., *et al.,* (1994). "Oral tolerance: Immunologic mechanisms and treatment of animal and human organ-specific autoimmune diseases by oral administration of autoantigens." *Annu. Rev. Immunol.* 12: 809–837.

314. Weiner, H.L. (1997). "Oral tolerance: Immune mechanisms and treatment of autoimmune diseases." *Immunol. Today* 7: 336–343.

314a. Osterholm, M., Schwartz, J. *Living Terrors* (Delacorte Press, 2000).

315. Rippon, S.W. *Medical Mycology* Third Edition (W. B. Saunders Company, 1988).

316. The News-Times, Dec. 2, 2001.

317. *USA Today* 5-15-02.

318. Pert, Candace. *Molecules of Emotion, The Science Behind Mind-Body Medicine* (Touchstone, 1999).

319. Ochman, James L. *Energy Medicine, The Scientific Basis* (Churchill Livingston, 2000).

320. New England School of Homeopathy, Seminars.

321. *Homeopathic News, Sept. 1892.*

322. *Investor's Business Daily,* Nov. 28, 1997.

323. Preston, Richard. *The Demon in the Freezer* (Random House, 2002).

324. "Persons with chronic conditions" (Nov. 13, 1996), *JAMA,* Vol. 276, No. 18.

325. "One Sick Country", *USA Today,* (June 28, 2001) based on a survey conducted by *The New England Journal of Medicine.*

326. Schmid, Ronald. *Native Nutrition: Eating According to Ancestral Wisdom* (Healing Arts Press, 1994).

327. Sears, Barry. *The Zone* (Regan Books, 1995).

328. Taubes, Gary. (July 7, 2002) "What if it's all been a big fat lie?" *The New York Times Magazine.*

329. Vimy, M.J., *et al.*, (1990) "Maternal-fetal distribution of mercury (203-Hg) released from dental amalgam fillings." *Am. J. Physiol.* 258, R939–R945.

330. Drasch, G., *et al.*, (1994) "Mercury burden of human fetal and infant tissues." *Eur. J. Pediat.* 153, 607–610.

331. Kuhnert P, *et al.*, (1981) "Comparison of Mercury levels in maternal blood fetal chord blood and placental tissue." *Am. J. Obstet. and Gynecol.*, 139:209–212.

332. Kuntz W.D., (1982) "Maternal and chord blood Mercury background levels; Longitudinal surveillance." *Am J Obstet and Gynecol.* 143:440–443.

333. Koos, *et al.*, (1976) "Mercury toxicity in pregnant women, fetus and newborn infant." *Am J Obstet And Gynecol.*, 126;390–409.

334. Khera, *et al.*, *Teratogenic and genetic effects of Mercury toxicity. The biochemistry of Mercury in the environment* (Nriagu, J.O. Ed Amsterdam Elsevier, 1979, 503–18).

335. Babich, *et al.*, (1985) "The mediation of mutagenicity and clastogenicity of heavy metals by physiochemical factors." Environ Res., 37;253–286.

336. *USA Today,* (Sept. 24, 2002) "Smallpox would face a massive response.".

337. *USA Today* (August 19, 2002) "U.S., Russia tussle over deadly anthrax sample.".

338. Clarke, John. *A Dictionary of Practical Materia Medica* (B. Jain publ. (P) Ltd., 1996)

339. Caduseus Institute of Classical Homeopathy Website, "Bioweapons and Homeopathy".

340. Lilienthal, Samuel. *Homoeopathic Therapeutics* (B. Jain Publishers (P) Ltd., 1996)

341. "Smallpox as a Biological Weapon" (June 9, 1999), *JAMA,* Vol. 281. No. 22.

342. Smith, Cyril W. *Electromagnetic Man: Health and Hazard in the Electrical Environment* (Simon Best, St. Martin's Press, Inc., November 1989)

343. Pert, Candace. *Molecules of Emotion, The Science Behind Mind-Body Medicine* (Simon and Schuster, 1999).

344. Kment, A. (1955) "Die Verteilung Trittium Markierung Herz, Leber, Nieren und Zellen bei alten Ratten." Die Therapiewoche. :152.

345. Wiener, Howard, et al., Science, (Feb. 1993, vol. 259, 26., p.p. 1321–1324).

346. Fukaura, Hi Koali, et al., Journ. of Clinical Investigation, vol. 98, #1, Jul. 1996.

347. Whitacre, Caroline, et al., (1996) "Oral tolerance. Mechanisms and Applications." vol. 778, Annals; NY Academy of Sciences, pp. 217–227.

348. Javeb, Najma, The Journal of Immunology (1995, vol. 155, pp. 1599–1605).

349. Santoro, Robert and Weyhreter, Alfred. (1993) "Support of Human/Organ Function with Raw Protein Concentrate as measure by Improvement in Serum Chemistry Values." J. of Applied Nutrition, vol. 45, #2.

350. "Cell infusion is a 'miracle' for diabetic" (May 12, 2002), USA Today.

351. Osband, M., et al., (1981) "Histiocytosis X—Demonstration of abnormal immunity, T cell Histamine H2 receptor deficiency and successful treatment with Thymic extract". New Engl. J. of Med., 304: 146–53.

352. Fiocchi, A., et al., (1986) "A double blind clinical trial for the evaluation of the therapeutical effectiveness of a calf thymus derivative (Thymomodulin) in children with recurrent respiratory infections." Thymus. 8:331.

353. Konmuro, K. & Bouse, E.A., (1973) "Induction of T-lymphocytes from precursor cells in vitro by a product of the thymus." Journal of Experimental Medicine. 138: 479–484.

354. Skotinicki, A. B. et al., "Biological properties and clinical use of calf thymus extract TFS-Polfa." In: Goldstein, A.L (ed), Thymic Hormones and Lymphokines. (New York City: Plenum Press, 1984), p.545.

355. Tas, M., et al., (June 1990) "Beneficial effects of the thymic hormone preparation Thymostimulin in patients with defects in cell-mediated immunity and chronic purulent rhinosinusitis. A double-blind cross-over trial on improvements in mono-

cyte polarization and clinical effects." *Clinical & Experimental Immunology:* 80(3):304.

356. Valesini, G., *et al.*, "A calf thymus lysate improves clinical symptoms and T-cell defects in the early stages of HIV infection: second report." *European Journal of Cancer and Clinical Oncology.* 23 :1915, 1987.

357. Martelli, M.F., *et al.*, (1982) "The in vivo effect of a thymus factor (Thymostimulin) on immunologic parameters of patients with untreated Hodgkin's disease." *Cancer* 50: 490.

358. Macchiarini, P., *et al.*, (Jan.–Feb. 1989) "Effects of Thymostimulinion chemotherapy-induced toxicity and longterm survival in small cell lung cancer patients." *Anticancer Research.* 9(1): 193.

359. Carrola, P., *et al.*, (1987) "In vivo modulating effect of calf thymus and lysate on human T-lymphocyte subsets and CD4 plus-CD8 plus ratio in the cause of different diseases." *Current Therapeutic Research.* 42: 1011–1017.

360. Ciconi, E., *et al.*, (May 1992) "Perioperative treatment with Thymostimulin in patients with stomach, and colorectal neoplasms. Our experience with 114 cases." *Minerva chirugica.* 47(10); 939.

361. Alba, E., *et al.*, (Dec 1991) "Prevention of infection and improvement of cenesthesia with Thymostimulin during chemotherapy following mastectomy." *Minerva Ginecologica.* 43(12):585.

362. Negi, L., *et al.*,(May 1992) "Chemotherapy and Thymostimulin in the treatment of advanced-stage breast neoplasma." *Minerva Medica.* 83(5); 283.

363. Martelli, M.F., *et al.*, (1982) "The in vivo effect of a thymus factor (Thymostimulin) on immunologic paramenters of patients with untreated Hodgkin's disease." *Cancer.* 50: 490)

364. Kaptchuk, Ted. *The Web That Has No Weaver* (Congdon and Weed, 1983).

365. Yunde H, Guoliang M., *et al.*, (1981) "Effect of Radix astraglis seuhedysari on the interferon system." *Chin Med J* 94:35–40.

366. German Ministry of Health, Echinesia Purpurea leaf. (1989)

Commission E. Monographs for Phytomedicines. Bonn, Germany: German Ministry of Health.

367. Scagline, F., *et al.*, (1990) "Immunomodulatory Effects of Two Extracts of Panax Ginseng C.A. Meyer." *Drugs Under Experimental Clinical Research* 16 no. 10: 537–542.

368. Yamamoto, M., Uemura, T., (1980) "Endocrinological and Metabolic Actions of P. Ginseng Principles." *Proceeding 3rd International Ginseng Symposium,* 15–119.

369. Bombardelli, E., Cirstoni, A., *et al.*, (1980) "The Effect of Acute and Chronic (Panax) Ginseng Saponins Treatment on Adrenal Function: Biochemical and Pharmacological." *Proceedings 3rd International Ginseng Symposium* 1, 9–16.

370. Fulder, S.J., (1981) "Ginseng and the Hypothalamic-Pituitary Control of Stress." *American Journal of Chinese Medicine* 9: 112–118.

371. Brekman, I. I., Dardymov, I.V., (1969) "Pharmacological Investigation of Glycosides From Ginseng and Eleutherococcus." *Lloydia* 32, 46–51.

372. Heiby, Walter. *The Reverse Effect How Vitamins and Minerals Promote Health and Cause Disease* (MediScience Publishers, 1988).

373. Flodin, NW. (1997) "The metabolic roles, pharmacology, and toxicology of lysine." *J Ar. Nutri,*16:7–21 (review).

374. Mender, Donald, M.D. *A Look at Paradoxes, Physics, and the Human Brain* (Plenum Press, 1994).

375. Kent, James. *Lectures on Homoeopathic Materia Medica* (B. Jain Publishers Pvt. Ltd., 1988)

376. Whitmont, Edward. *Psyche and Substance* (North Atlantic Books).

377. Coulter, Catherine. *Portraits of Homeopathic Medicines* (Quality Medical Publishing, Inc.)

378. *USA Today,* March 28, 2002.

379. *Homeopathy Today,* Jan. 2002, Vol. 22 #1.

380. Gray, Bill. *Homeopathy—Science or Myth* (North Atlantic Books, Berkeley, 2000)

381. Ullman, Dana (1999) "Homeopathy and Managed Care: Manageable or Unmanageable", *Journal of Alternative and Complementary Medicine.*

382. Caisse Nationale de l'Assurance Maladie des Travailleurs Salaris, 1996.

383. Sharples F, van Haselen, R. "Patients perspective on using a complementary medicine approach to their health." (a survey at the Royal London Homeopathic Hospital NHS Trust).

384. HomInform, Homoeopathy: The Guide (CDRom), June, 1, 1997.

385. Swayne J. (Jul. 1992) "The cost and effectiveness of homeopathy." *British Homoeopathic Journal,* 81, 3:148–150.

386. Gerhard I, *et al.,*(1991) "Weibliche fertiltitasstorungen. Vergleich homoopa.thischer einzelmittel—mit konventioneller hormontherapie." Therapeutikon. 7:309–315.

387. Jacobs J., Smith N. (Nov. 18–21, 1996) "Charges, utilization, and practice patterns from a pilot insurance program covering alternative medical services." American Public Health Association Conference, New York City.

388. Jonas W.B., Jacobs J. *Healing with Homeopathy.* (New York, Warner, 1996).

389. Ullman, D. *Homeopathy: Medicine for the 21st Century* (North Atlantic Books, Berkeley, 1991a).

390. Gray, William. *Homeopathy—Science or Myth* (North Atlantic Books, Berkeley, 2000)

391. *Banner of Light,* March 12, 1898.

392. Coulter, Harris L. *Divided Legacy: The Conflict Between Homoeopathy and the American Medical Association* (North Atlantic Books, 1973, 1982).

393. Transactions of the New York State Homeopathic Medical Society, 1867.

394. JAMA, 1872.

395. Duffin, Jacalyn. *History of Medicine* (Toronto University of Toronto Press, 1999)

396. *Journal of the American Institute of Homeopathy,* V (1912–1913), 1352. *Proceedings of the House of Delegates of the American Medical Association,* 1913, 2, 50; 1914, 3–4, 46. American Medical Association, *Digest of Official Actions, 1846–1958,* 148.

397. Coulter, Harris L. *Divided Legacy: The Conflict Between Ho-*

moeopathy and the American Medical Association (North Atlantic Books, 1973, 1982).

398. Ibid.
399. Miller, Monica. (Summer 2002) "Pharmacists cash-in and sell-out homeopathy", *Innovation.*
400. *"Persons with chronic conditions",* Nov. 13, 1996, *JAMA,* Vol. 276, No. 18.
401. "Finger pointers can't settle on who's to blame for health costs", *USA Today,* August 21, 2002.
402. Ibid.
403. *The Wall Street Journal,* 3-21-02.
404. Reilly, David Taylor. (July 30, 1993), *"Young Doctors' Views on Alternative Medicine",* British Medical Journal, 287, 337–339.
405. Wharton, R., Lewith, G. (1996) "Complementary Medicine and the General Practitioner." *Brit. Med. J.* 292:1498.
406. British Institute of Homeopathy News, International; No. 63, 2002.
407. Fisher, P., Ward, A. (1994) Complementary Medicine in Europe. *Brit. Med. J.* 309:107)
408. Bellavite, P., Signorini, A. (1995) *Homeopathy—A Frontier in Medical Science,* (North Atlantic *Books,* 1995, p. 271–272).
409. Jonas, W., Jacobs, J. *Healing with Homeopathy.* (Warner Books, New York, 1996).
410. Ibid.
411. Bellavite, P., Signorini, A. *The Emerging Science of Homeopathy: Complexity, Biodynamics, and Nanopharmacology* (North Atlantic Books, February 2002)
412. Ibid.
413. Ramakrishnan, Dr. A.U., Coulter, Catherine R. *A Homeopathic Approach to Cancer,* (Quality Medical Publishing, 2001)
414. Bellavite, P., Signorini, A. *The Emerging Science of Homeopathy: Complexity, Biodynamics, and Nanopharmacology* (North Atlantic Books, February 2002).
415. Eizayaga, Francisco X. "Homeopathy in American-Spanish-Speaking Countries" A Presentation at the Annual Conference of the National Center for Homeopathy, Oct. 4–5 1995.

416. World Homeopathic Directory (New Delhi: Harjeet, 1982), pp. 36–37; Eizayaga, "Homeopathy".

417. Jonas, W., Jacobs, J. *Healing with Homeopathy,* (Warner Books).

418. Resolution A4-0075, 1997.

419. Scholten, Jan. *Homeopathy and the Elements* (Stichting Alonnissos, 1996).

420. Burton Goldberg Group. *Alternative Medicine: The Definite Guide* (Future Medicine Publishing, Inc., 1994).

421. Berman B., *et al.,* (July 1997) "Homeopathy and the US primary care physician." *British Homoeopathic Journal.* 86:131–138.

422. "Selling Shyness", *New Republic,* August 2, 1999.

423. "Feds warn drugmakers: gifts to doctors may be illegal", *USA Today,* Oct. 2, 2002.

424. "Drug firms and doctors: the offers pour in", *Boston Globe,* December 15, 2002.

425. Miller, Monica. " Pharmacists cash-in and sell-out homeopathy", *Innovation,* Summer 2002.

426. U.S. House of Representatives Committee on Government Reform Hearings: "Comprehensive Medical Care for Bioterrorism Exposure—Are We Making Evidence-Based Decisions? What Are the Research Needs?", November, 2001.

Index

Appendix

The recommended book list for the serious reader

1. *The Emerging Science of Homeopathy: Complexity, Biodynamics, and Nanopharmacology,* Paolo Bellavite, Andrea Signorini, February 2002, North Atlantic Books.
2. *Fundamental Research in Ultra High Dilution and Homoeopathy,* Jurgen Schulte, Peter Christian Endler, May 1998, Kluwer Academic Publishers.
3. *Signals and Images,* Madeleine Bastide, March 1997, Kluwer Academic Publishers.
4. *Science and Human Transformation: Subtle Energies, Intentionality and Consciousness,* William A. Tiller, August 1997, Pavior Publishing.
5. *Conscious Acts of Creation—The Emergence of a New Physics,* William A. Tiller, Walter E. Dibble, Michael J. Kohane, October 2001, Pavior Publishing.
6. *Electromagnetic Man: Health and Hazard in the Electrical Environment,* Cyril W. Smith, Simon Best, November 1989, St. Martin's Press, Inc.
7. *Power vs. Force,* Hawkins, David R., 1995, Veritas Publishing

For Educational Events and Learning Resources contact :

"SYY Integrated Health Systems, Ltd.",
37 King Street
Chappaqua, New York 10514
phone: (914) 861-9161
e-mail: *seminar@yurkovsky.com*
website: *www.yurkovsky.com*

About the Author

Dr. Yurkovsky received his M.D. degree from II Moscow State Medical Institute, in the former USSR, in 1975. He completed his Internal Medicine Residency and Fellowship in Cardiovascular Medicine at Coney Island Hospital of Downstate Medical School, Brooklyn, New York and is Board Certified in Internal Medicine. He is a former or current member of many professional organizations including the American College of Advancement in Medicine (ACAM), American Institute of Homeopathy, and is also one of the founding directors along with Dr. Robert Atkins and other alternative physicians of Foundation for the Advancement of Innovative Medicine (FAIM) in New York.

Disenchanted with the dismal yield of conventional medicine in the care of chronic diseases, he turned to the exploration and thorough study of Alternative Medicine. Having realized that the primary source of health and disease, according to physics, stem from the corresponding cellular energy fields, he adopted a new revolutionary medical model, one that interfaces the theories of biology and physics, established by his mentor, Professor Emeritus of Materials Science, William A. Tiller, of Stanford University. Based on this model, Dr. Yurkovsky has determined diagnostic and therapeutic priorities for the successful integration of various alternative and conventional approaches. This has led him to transform the often vague nature of medical specialties from "hit and miss" paradigms into a far more effective, exact and predictable science. Dr. Yurkovsky has, also, founded his own teaching institution, *"SYY Integrated Health Systems, Ltd.,"* which is dedicated to sharing his medical system under the concept of FCT—Field Control Therapy®. Since 1999, he has taught this curriculum to medical doctors and licensed health care professionals with special emphasis on energy-based diagnostic and therapeutic modalities aimed particularly at toxicological, biological and nuclear agents. These, as a rule, elude conventional diagnostic methods, yet represent the primary source of chronic diseases in patients.

Part of this curriculum has been also dedicated to the medical management of biological, chemical and nuclear warfare. In the fall of 2000, almost a year before September 11, he called on the National Security Council under the White House to draw their attention to the methods presented in detail in this book.

Dr. Yurkovsky resides with his wife and two children in Connecticut, and maintains a private practice in Chappaqua, New York.